THE CYCLE BOOK

The
Cycle Book

An Interactive Step-by-Step Guide to Tracking Hormones and Knowing Your Body

Laura Federico, MSW, LCSW, CST
Morgan Miller, CPM, LM, IBCLC

A TarcherPerigee Book

tarcherperigee

an imprint of Penguin Random House LLC
1745 Broadway, New York, NY 10019
penguinrandomhouse.com

TarcherPerigee with tp colophon is a registered trademark of Penguin Random House LLC

Most TarcherPerigee books are available at special quantity discounts for bulk purchase for sales promotions, premiums, fundraising, and educational needs. Special books or book excerpts also can be created to fit specific needs. For details, write SpecialMarkets@penguinrandomhouse.com.

Library of Congress Cataloging-in-Publication Data
has been applied for.

Trade paperback ISBN: 9780593717059
Ebook ISBN: 9780593717066

Printed in the United States of America
1st Printing

Book design by Shannon Nicole Plunkett

The authorized representative in the EU for product safety and compliance is Penguin Random House Ireland, Morrison Chambers, 32 Nassau Street, Dublin D02 YH68, Ireland, https://eu-contact.penguin.ie.

Dedicated to our clients

Contents

Foreword

I typed and retyped the text for weeks, always deleting it before pressing send. Morgan and I had been friends since our early twenties when we were living piled on top of one another in a string of tiny Brooklyn apartments. But now, over a decade later, what I needed from Morgan felt like too much, and I felt so broken that it took me months to ask. I knew how busy she was, and as with all our friends in a helping profession—in her case, midwifery—I felt ashamed that I was about to ask her to clock in. As a clinical sex therapist, I felt I should have been able to solve this type of problem myself.

The official diagnosis was unexplained secondary infertility. So far, I had followed the pathway laid out for me by my doctors. I took the fertility medications that would stimulate my hormones to facilitate "super ovulation," even after expressing my worries about the medication and putting in a good word for my non-super, yet regular, ovulation. I came in once a month so the nurses could use a catheter to send washed sperm directly into my uterus, a process known as intra-uterine insemination (IUI). (And also to find a way to pay the clinic large sums of money not covered by my insurance.)

I felt my body get almost immediately sick from the fertility medication. After multiple past attempts to treat premenstrual dysphoric disorder (PMDD) with different hormonal birth control pills and strategically timed selective serotonin reuptake inhibitors (SSRIs), I had learned that my body and mind were dramatically impacted by hormonal shifts. When I voiced my concerns to my providers, they told me that what I had were normal side effects. When I became clinically depressed and stopped bleeding entirely, they only rarely returned my phone calls. "This happens," they said.

When I asked how I could get pregnant when my body was so sick, when I had stopped bleeding, and when I felt certain I had stopped ovulating, they told me to stick with the fertility medications. In my conversations with my providers, there were no other options. As instructed, I would go to the office once a month, after I would pee on the ovulation test preferred by my doctor and a smiley face appeared. My body didn't feel like I was ovulating when I saw this cartoon smile, but I would go in anyway, crying every time I arrived and every time I left. I felt so far from myself, but I hoped that the doctors knew my body better than I did.

Finally, I texted Morgan because I just couldn't go back to that clinic.

Morgan responded immediately and did in fact "clock in." She went over my paperwork from multiple doctors, taught me proper cycle tracking, reviewed my data, validated my own body awareness—and supported my choice to discontinue the fertility medications. She also referred me to an acupuncturist who, astoundingly, was the first provider in this entire saga to ask me exploratory questions about my menstrual cycles.

It was during my quest to find a new fertility practice, reaching out to multiple specialists, armed with my tracking data, and going to weekly acupuncture, that I connected with a doctor who advertised a diversity of infertility interventions. When meeting any new provider, I felt pressure to show up in a way that might compel them to take me seriously. I delivered my rehearsed story, presented the information I had from tracking and previous fertility testing, and tried not to be "too emotional."

He too dismissed me, telling me that I needed to track using a system specific to his practice for a minimum of six months before being seen again and that I was also required to take classes to learn the system. I politely pushed back, trying not to take up too much space—couldn't he see that I had been tracking the same things as his system? I had the information he was looking for already! As I was on my way out, not successful in holding back my tears, he glanced at my paperwork and asked if he could refer patients to me for psychological treatment. "I've noticed that people seem to have a really hard time with this process. I never have enough therapists to refer to—they are always full."

Morgan and my acupuncturist helped me reconnect with my body, with whom I previously felt at war. I needed to be present with it in order to begin making choices for my care. Tracking reestablished a sense of trust in myself, a feeling that I had some agency. Tracking supported the belief that I could take care of myself. This felt like a truth I could return to after a difficult appointment, a reminder of what I could handle.

It would take many more meetings before I found a reproductive endocrinologist who listened to me. It took many more months to heal from the impact of the fertility medications, to start bleeding and ovulating again, and longer to believe that there was nothing wrong with my cycle, my sexuality, or my body.

Many of the people I work with come to therapy because they too have been told there is something inexplicably wrong with them. The limited options they have been given don't seem to be working and don't feel like the right fit. Their experience with their sexuality isn't represented in the mainstream discourse, and their well-meaning friends don't know what to say. The people I work with know themselves but must fight shame, stigma, and a one-size-fits-all approach to be able to fully take care of themselves.

It is clear to me now that there is nothing broken about me and that there are many ways to work with one's body when something doesn't feel right. The infertility treatments that are the right fit for so many were simply not the best fit for me.

Morgan and I haven't lived in the same place in a long time, but our friendship has survived the distance. During a long-overdue vacation (after Morgan had given me a quick ultrasound on the couch of our Airbnb), I asked her if she might be interested in working on this project with me. Because almost two years after my experience at the clinic, I had conceived after my first try of IUI without fertility medications.

We wrote this book to be a part of the fight for a return to bodily agency. To offer a tool in the process of ownership over well-being. The experience of self-advocacy in our current social and medical system requires immense emotional labor. Our hope is that the framework laid out here offers some respite in the ongoing struggle to be treated as experts over our own bodies.

LAURA FEDERICO

With my first menstrual cycles, I remember quietly celebrating the cramps as a rite into adulthood, but it didn't take long before those cramps became debilitating, and my pride was overpowered by pain. Soon each cycle felt like someone was pouring acid into my abdomen and wringing my intestines like a wet rag. My mother reassured me that her periods had been this way, as her mother's had been before her, and she shared her family line of coping techniques. She said learning to cope with the pain would aid me in labor one day. For years, for about three days every cycle, I would try to convince myself I wasn't dying.

Inevitably this cyclic pain interrupted my day-to-day teenage life. My doctor also told me that my experience was normal and treated me with a few high-dose painkillers before settling on the birth control pill. I was elated to find that the magic little pill worked like a charm and my period pain could now be managed through an easily obtained prescription. My thoughts became once again occupied by school and enormous teenage feelings, no longer distracted by pain. It was lifesaving.

I lived with this manageable pain well into my late twenties, loving my birth control pill for all the reasons it was created. You can imagine my shock, then, at twenty-six years old, when I found out I was pregnant. Emotionally, I felt that the pill had betrayed me, and I made the complex decision to schedule an abortion.

I arrived at the clinic feeling nervous but well-informed about what was going to take place: ultrasound, bloodwork, and scheduling the procedure. Then the ultrasound technician told me that I needed to go straight to the emergency room across town. That was it, no further information than that the pregnancy did not appear as it should. I fell into a panic, followed their directions, and was then transferred between three facilities for two weeks before resolving the pregnancy.

In the end, I was so overwhelmed with the relief of no longer being pregnant that I gratefully headed home and didn't look back. For me, the pill had not effectively prevented pregnancy even when taken correctly, but they assured me that my newly placed hormonal intrauterine device (IUD) was even better. I would cramp and spot for three months, they added. My provider recommended I get black underwear.

Months went by, and that ever-familiar pain in my abdomen crept back in. My doctor prescribed me narcotics and muscle relaxants, but even those didn't seem to do much. Reluctantly, I decided to remove the IUD and return to my jilted love, the pill, for its pain relief. A few weeks later, while trying on clothes in a fitting room, I felt a sharp pain in my inner leg, and I noticed an alarming black and red bruise striping my inner thigh. I touched it and it felt like a hot stick was implanted under my skin. I went to my doctor only to once again be sent straight to the emergency room. I was diagnosed with thrombophlebitis, also known as blood clots. The doctor asked me two questions: "Do you have a family history of blood clots? How long have you been on hormonal birth control?" Yes, and nearly fifteen years. His response: "You shouldn't take that anymore."

That ER doctor explained how my body had been responding to long-term hormonal therapy. He explained that the pill had been a great option for my pain relief initially, but with my given history, it was not a forever treatment plan. Suddenly I could backtrack the aches and pains I'd ignored over the years. My body had been communicating with me the entire time, but I simply hadn't been taught my body's language to understand what it was trying to say. While my severe cramping had nearly stopped, I began to understand that hormonal birth control was treating my symptoms but hadn't been treating the underlying cause: endometriosis.

Later on, I realized my traumatic abortion experience could have been different. The ultrasound technician had been fearful I was experiencing an ectopic pregnancy, a pregnancy that would potentially require emergency surgery. Unfortunately, within the healthcare shuffle, that information and the resolution of my emergent status was never communicated to me.

As a teen, if I'd been told I wasn't a candidate for hormonal birth control, maybe I wouldn't have ended up back in the ER a second time, dealing with blood clots, and maybe I would have received my endometriosis diagnosis earlier. Had an ectopic pregnancy been explained to me—including that it was ruled out with follow-up ultrasounds—maybe the whole experience wouldn't have felt so scary. I would have had the opportunity to engage with that process in a way that felt grounded and affirming rather than coping by disassociating and trying to forget.

These maybes led me to a career devoted to listening to people's experiences with their bodies. They led me to sharing tools on how to learn each language an individual's body speaks. These maybes led me into becoming a midwife. These maybes led me to *The Cycle Book*.

Over the years, Laura and I have acted as clinical consultants for one another's private practices and steadily complained about *this thing* that didn't exist, this way of connecting modalities and offering people agency. Laura proposed we make it, make *this thing* that didn't exist. Without hesitation, I was in.

MORGAN MILLER

THE CYCLE BOOK

1.

Introducing a Model of Tracking for Everyone

"I feel invisible."

"It's like I was just a number to them."

The people we work with say this. We've felt this ourselves.

We are rendered invisible every day through the lack of prioritization and education of our bodies.

Most of us just haven't been taught to be aware of our bodies. In fact, we've been trained to actively ignore our body's signals for so long that we don't know which way is up.

Cycle tracking is a direct pathway to reclaiming ownership over our bodies. Most people believe this process is a simple record of bleeding, but in our work, we have seen the transformative power of a far deeper method.

Tracking has largely been relegated to the realm of people trying to get pregnant, where it can be a frustrating experience that feels like homework. It's safe to say that menstruation, vastly understudied and discussed primarily in the context of reproduction, has not been given its due by science and culture. It comes, then, as no surprise that the tools we have to understand it in ourselves are similarly reductive and limited in scope. We've been done wrong! The revolutionary tool of tracking is so valuable that it demands democratization. Tracking should be made available to and used by *everyone*.

This model is about way more than paying attention to when you bleed. This is much bigger than that. It's about connection; it's expansive. It is not just about fertility. This is not just about hormones. It's not even just about connecting with your overall health. Cycle tracking provides you with connections to all of those experiences and more. It gives you the ability to identify and place those connections in the context of your surroundings, environment, world, universe . . . We're talking from the minute detail to the great big picture of it all. But this model of tracking is not being shared and we are not being taught how to listen to our bodies.

And so, in our work as a clinical sex therapist and a licensed midwife, we've heard over and over that "nobody told me this," and we have been left with the same outrage and dismay as our clients.

It is this disservice that drove us to create this tracking system—a model designed to assist us all in recognizing, recording, and making sense of anything we might be experiencing in our bodies and minds. When we say *anything*, we really mean it. In fact, hormonal fluctuations are directly linked to changes in mental health, cognition, pain, sexuality, the metabolic system, chronic health conditions, sleep, and so much more.

THE REASON WE'RE HERE

Who is this book for? If you're looking to expand the pleasure in your life, we can help with that. Is pain interfering with the important things? Tracking can help you manage and prevent it. Looking to be better able to regulate your moods and emotions? We are here to help you to learn so much about yourself and find increased attention and clarity about feelings, thoughts, and emotions. Do you feel uncomfortable in your body? We will guide you through it. Have you felt dismissed when seeking medical support or that you haven't been treated with care? Does sex hurt? Following your cycle can help, and if you know something's wrong but don't yet have a diagnosis, this process might help you to get there sooner. Want to better understand a relationship in your life? You can. If you've recently started menstruating, this process can be invaluable. The same goes for perimenopause and everything in between.

Here's the thing: There's nothing too big or too small to track. There's no right or wrong way to track.

Millions of people track their cycles on apps, but those apps are also tracking you—sometimes in ways that are not legal or consensual—and they for sure don't go deep enough. Tracking apps leave users vulnerable to surprisingly inaccurate fertility predictions, with some studies estimating their efficacy at about 20 percent for correctly predicting ovulation. And in the United States, in this post-Roe era, many privacy and health advocates recommend that we delete our tracking apps entirely because although they collect sensitive health information, this information is usually not protected. Current U.S. federal privacy laws were designed to primarily protect health information shared between doctors, healthcare facilities, and insurers, and so data mining has been able to proliferate as we wait for policy to adapt. We need to protect ourselves by protecting our data— and getting it out of the cloud and down on paper is one way to do that.

We've spent years cultivating the most effective ways to help the people we work with understand their patterns and arm themselves with useful information to guide their one-of-a-kind treatments. Confronted with the difficulties so many of us have with simply being aware of our bodies, we have created accessible methods for you to listen to yourself and feel safe.

Tracking fosters trust. It allows you to know yourself, to believe in yourself, and to begin to heal from all the times that other people made the choices about your body *for* you.

Clients come to us all the time feeling broken, saying things like "My body has failed me." They've seen multiple providers and no one has been able to "fix them." This is the language of the oppressor. Things happening in your body may require attention, care, or medical intervention; this does *not* mean your body is broken. Instead, they often point to the body or the mind asking for new and different support systems. You are perfect, even if you are experiencing a painful condition, feeling frustrated and disconnected from yourself. When we are in pain, in whatever way it is manifesting, it is often our mind or body communicating with us to make changes. The thing that isn't perfect and is broken and does need fixing isn't us; it's the systems around us.

Every day in our respective practices, we have seen how a more comprehensive understanding of our body and cycles can transform the way we see—and speak for—ourselves. We regularly see amazing direct benefits from this process. As we create your personal tracking journey together, you can expect:

Confidence and comfort with your body and being

Healing from medical, sexual, and systemic trauma

Pain prevention and management

A greater knowledge of your body and yourself and ways to support it and you

Increased attention and clarity about feelings, thoughts, and emotions

An expansion of pleasure in your life

This is the wild thing about tracking: it can heal you when you didn't even realize you needed to be healed.

YOU'RE IN CHARGE

It might be hard to believe that you can be in charge when many of us live in environments that work tirelessly to strip us of our bodily agency. When we live in countries where our rights to abortion, birth control, and bodily choice are evaporating in front of our eyes. When we advocate for ourselves to a healthcare system, only to be ignored, talked down to, or mistreated. When our law enforcement and legal systems blame us for the violence that happens to us. When the culture around us does not protect us against abuses of power and sexual assault. When the language we need to understand our bodies is actively withheld from us as an act of erasure.

How can we be the experts when the world around us claims knowledge and power over our bodies?

We are here to remind you that you're in charge.

You deserve full agency to understand, advocate for, and determine what to do with your body. And despite what you might have been told by loved ones, strangers, or even healthcare providers, you and you alone deserve the final say when it comes to your body.

This book was born out of our shared frustrations with the lack of resources available for people who want to know and exercise agency over their bodies. We've worked with many clients who have been left without the resources they needed to understand an emotion or a sensation and were instead bombarded with messages about what they "should" be feeling—or dismissed altogether.

At times, personal and systemic abuses of power may prevent you from accessing your agency. Maybe you have had choices made for you—choices you did not ask for and did not consent to. Reclaiming a feeling of agency and choice can help. Finding this within the body is a way forward, and through tracking, a sense of power is accessible.

We've dedicated our personal and professional lives—and now, this book—to listening to what bodies are communicating and to combating some of the sociocultural influences that disrupt that communication. We've focused not only on recognizing what's happening in our bodies and minds but also on identifying the cycles these sensations flow through. This book arms you with data to use in any way you want and to advocate for yourself in any part of your life.

YOU DESERVE TO BE TAKEN CARE OF

We've got to switch it up. The current conversation around cycle tracking is largely medicalized, gendered, and heteronormative. This leaves many people out of the conversation altogether. This reductive, fertility-focused lens has altered the broader scope around menstruation, hormonal shifts, and the body. We're viewing our bodies and ourselves in an incomplete manner. We're ignoring how interconnected our body systems are and how cyclic hormones interplay in all levels of being.

A twenty-eight-day cycle length does not apply to the vast majority of people who menstruate, and cycle variability is influenced by a huge number of factors, including stress, social dynamics, life responsibilities, and sleep. Plus, cycle-to-cycle changes are normal and to be expected.

Identifying your unique hormonal cycle can illuminate your overall body functioning and feeling. Cycle tracking can even identify patterns that are totally unrelated to hormones and may be a result of life events. Vast awareness of the body and the mind is available through tracking. Understanding your cycle can even be the missing link to getting a chronic illness diagnosis or the final piece of the puzzle in understanding your mental health.

You deserve to be taken care of and you are perfect.

That's truly it. We say this to every person we work with. And pretty much everyone we know. And the thing is, we believe it. When either of us says this to a client for the first time, you can see the surprise etched on their face. They usually don't say a thing. Sometimes they laugh. But the more we say it, the more you can see they also start to believe it.

And, little by little, they're not surprised anymore.

No one can define, feel, or articulate the nuance of your existence better than you. Not a single person, machine, or algorithm can do that to the level of complexity that you can. By merely being in your body you will always know more about your body than any other expert in any other field.

If you take away anything from this book, we hope it is this:

You are the expert of your body.

SOME WAYS TO USE CYCLE TRACKING

At its core, this book is here to help you track the patterns within your body and mind, which can open a powerful pathway to self-understanding. You're able to take the information you gather and ask a vital but often overlooked question: "How do I want to take care of myself?" Prioritizing the mindful practice of self-observation can be both powerful and pleasurable.

Use your *Cycle Book* to:

Create an invaluable repository of data
Cycle tracking allows you to learn the things that sex education likely failed to

teach you. It helps you gain greater awareness and understanding of your bodily sensations, recognize the connections between your body and mind, and learn things about your parts, feelings, needs, and desires. This data can be used in those difficult and vulnerable moments when it's hard to articulate our needs.

Identify when something doesn't feel right

The menstrual cycle can act as a signifier of overall health and an early communicator when other systems in your body are overwhelmed. Cycle analysis uncovers information about far more than bleeding. Like checking in on heart rate, body temperature, respiratory rate, or blood pressure, your menstrual cycle is a window into the way your body is functioning.

Use mindful self-awareness to feel better

Cycle tracking is the process of compassionately listening to yourself and tapping into your feelings. A regular prioritization of the whole self is a crucial piece of finding comfort and ease in our bodies. With an attention to curiosity and an explicit lack of pressure around outcome, just observing the body is an act of care. Throughout this book we use the mindfulness skill of *non-judgmental awareness*. We practice body neutrality and embodied safety to be present with your body, even when it's tough. There is pleasure in the practice of gaining awareness of your body.

Enhance communication with yourself and others

Hormonal cycles can affect your whole being, including how you relate to others. Learning your cycle trends can allow you to set up structures of engagement that align to you. Shifting the way you interact with those in your orbit to reflect what feels most affirming based on your state of being can impact all those relationships. This strengthens communication with yourself; intimate, romantic, and sexual partners; and family, friends, colleagues, and acquaintances.

Facilitate self-advocacy within greater healthcare systems

Your recorded data about your thoughts, feelings, and bodily sensations can help your healthcare provider (be it a primary care physician, gynecologist, midwife, psychotherapist, psychiatrist, physical therapist, or any other provider) get a bigger, broader picture of what you're experiencing. It can inform clinical decisions and guide collaborative care. Without this information, providers may only be able to treat a particular symptom instead of understanding how and why other systems in the body may be involved. Cycle tracking can also guide you and your healthcare provider in making decisions about how certain supplements or medications can impact your body.

Realize that you are not alone

We know how lonely it can feel when things get difficult in your body. We are here with you every step of the way. There are so many other people out in the world learning to listen to their bodies, learning about how to take care of—and advocate for—themselves and others. This is a community.

YOUR DATA IS YOURS

In this book, we recognize any and all reasons one might want to track their cycle—as well as every person's right to bodily privacy and autonomy. For many communities, tracking bodily data like a menstrual cycle hasn't always been accessible, and in recent years that data has been bought and sold without explicit consent or, in extreme cases, legally used against those who have tracked it.

In a cultural moment when our data is being weaponized, this book is a tool that enables you to be in control of your bodily privacy and to learn about the cyclical sensations you might be feeling.

Our goal for this book is to provide you with a forum to:

Explore the relationships between your mind and body

Record any sensations you're experiencing

Be in control of your own data

Connect with your pleasure

Find your own unique normal

Learning your body is like learning a new language. At first, it's tricky. Four years of taking French and all you can pronounce is *croissant*. New languages are hard. Your individual body's language, though, is gorgeous. It's different and it's only yours. You're the best expert of this language in the entire universe. No one else knows more of it than you. *The Cycle Book* will guide you into fluency and easy conversation, so much so that at some point you won't even have to consciously translate this language. You'll know it so well you'll dream in it.

2.

How This Book Is Organized

This book is yours. A good chunk is designated for your personal pattern-tracking and pattern-recognition system. Over time, you'll fill in these pages with the knowledge you'll gain about yourself—body and mind. In the middle you'll find blank charts ready for your use. Take a glance at pages 135–165 if you'd like to visualize some of these charts in use as you move through this book.

To start us out, chapter 3, "Tracking Defined," explores how this method might be different than cycle tracking you've seen before and defines the simple steps involved. Years of work in midwifery and psychology informed this set of data collection queries.

Chapter 4, "Interconnected Self," explores the established links between mind and body and includes a discussion around ways to get curious about possible personal connections. Prompts guide you in understanding how your hormones might impact your physical, emotional, sexual, cognitive, and relational self. Further guided exploration provides you with your own bank of tracking-ready individualized categories for use with charting.

There are *tracking prep guides* throughout this book. These interactive journal exercises allow us to walk with you as you delve into identifying the thoughts, emotions, and physical feelings that you will ultimately decide to track. Doing this prep work will maximize your charting. A combination of clinical and emotional, these guides incorporate mindfulness and body-based perspectives, interventions that have been shown to be especially useful in increasing awareness of our own bodies and improving our health outcomes.

In chapter 5, "Pleasure," we advocate for an inclusion of experiences that feel good to you. Beyond an invitation to bring pleasure into your daily experience, this chapter identifies the transformative power of tracking pleasure. We build on the science behind the benefits of self-compassion and care. Tracking pleasure can create pleasure.

In chapter 6, "Safety," using a warm and acceptance-based approach, we work with you to define your self-regulation systems. A combination of evidence-based clinical mindfulness and somatic perspectives provide the foundation for guided exercises. We focus on using your strengths to take care of yourself and your body. Concrete tools are included for use in grounding and regulating yourself while coping with difficult experiences.

In chapter 7, "Dissociation," we highlight the protective nature of responses that are designed to assist in survival and explore how these responses can impact cycles and sensation tracking. The factors of big-*T* and small-*t* trauma interfere with people's ability to feel safe in their bodies and take care of themselves and their hormonal cycles. In this chapter, we share our favorite practical tools for living with trauma, showcasing ways you can safely and comfortably be present in your body and track sensations. We explain a relevant post-traumatic response—dissociation—that many of us are familiar with.

In chapter 8, "Pain," the body's suffering is validated and measured. Maybe your pain has been dismissed before. Not here. We explore implicit bias in the medical system, medical research, and society. We tackle pelvic, genital, and hormonally related pain conditions with compassion. You are given direct and actionable resources to identify, track, and connect with support to manage any pain you might have. Pain is one of the more common presenting concerns for those seeking support in tracking. In response, this chapter is appropriately robust, providing a list of genital and pelvic pain conditions that often take multiple visits to multiple doctors to get diagnosed (if ever officially diagnosed). This list is based on research as well as the experiences of our work in our clinics. An inclusive and descriptive pain scale is introduced to more accurately track your experience.

Chapter 9, "Cycle Phases," is an accessible take on the phases of the menstrual cycle, including bleeding, the follicular phase, ovulation, and the luteal phase. We explore the signs of each phase, how to identify them, what each might mean for your body, and how to track them.

Chapter 10, "Hormones," explores how hormonal messengers regulate our bodies throughout our lives. This is not only a breakdown of the significant hormonal players but a comprehensive look at how they directly show up in a person's mind and body on a day-to-day basis. Understanding these hormones unlocks possibilities for care. We go beyond sex hormones, as we know that cyclical hormones interplay with other body and hormonal systems. We give you tools to identify how the major hormones might be impacting your body and mind.

Chapter 13, "Your Cycle Patterns," explains the many ways your data can be interpreted and used to feel better and guides you through a simple step-by-step process to identify your cycle patterns.

In chapter 14, "Anatomy," we define and explain the relevant body systems, emphasizing that every body is different and that anatomy can change over time and with certain hormonal shifts. We identify body parts for what they are. We expand the traditional "reproductive" anatomy to include all greater body systems, which are also impacted by hormonal cycles. Turns out not everything about your uterus has to do with reproducing. Reference this chapter at any time!

In chapter 15, "Body Fluids," we explore fluids you might notice during your cycle, identifying what they might mean and how to check for them. These body fluids are also often referred to as cervical fluids or discharge. This chapter provides observation options that reflect different levels of comfort and access. We challenge the traditional hierarchical method of observation and give you tools to observe your own body fluids in ways that are good for *you*. This is a core component to successful tracking, and many people have not received education around how to notice and interpret body fluids. Gentle and encouraging, this chapter provides critical sex ed while also giving you choices over your relationship with your body. We provide context around stigma and ways to combat it.

Chapter 16, "Basal Body Temperature (BBT)," explains why measuring your resting temperature is so critical and how you can use this measurement to gain insight into your body's hormonal shifts. BBT tracking is one of the simplest ways to visualize how your body processes and uses hormones like estrogen and progesterone. Our charts use a simplified version of daily temperature collection to maximize the impact of this task.

Chapter 17, "Birth Control," explores how to track while using different forms of birth control. We discuss tracking when transitioning on or off birth control as well as the hormonal impacts of being on different types.

Chapter 18, "Fertility Choices," touches on the complexities of the subject and the ways in which we can broaden this discussion to include individual and collective well-being. This tracking is for readers making sure they do not conceive, those wanting to conceive, those not sure if they want to conceive, those experiencing challenges conceiving, and those who have lost a pregnancy. Common tests are explained and contextualized. We treat this topic kindly and neutrally and detail common difficulties you might encounter.

In chapter 19, "Perimenopause," we level up in understanding this phase of life that brings significant hormonal change, walk through the symptoms you might experience, and explore how tracking can help you better manage these sensations. Perimenopause can last up to fifteen years. This topic remains underdiscussed, and this chapter explicitly details and a broad list of sensations related to this life phase.

You are the expert on you. We conclude with the offer of one final resource to center you and your priorities if you are engaging with health providers.

We share many stories, too. These are based on real experiences of real people we have been lucky enough to work with throughout the years. Their stories have been anonymized and combined to illustrate the body's journey while keeping their identities protected. We meet with people both briefly and for many years and we have always upheld and will continue to uphold their confidentiality.

Use this book in whatever way works for you. Read cover-to-cover, skim certain sections, or spend your time solely on the tracking exercises.

When we were writing and designing this book, our goal was for pleasure to be a priority. So often, pleasure is either ignored or considered off-limits, and rarely is it seen as relevant to the menstrual cycle. Our educational system's emphasis on the outcome of bodily functions means that many of us haven't been taught to understand how those functions might feel. And we certainly haven't been taught how to feel good. In our prioritization of this new framework for well-being, we suggest that pleasure could be infused into any part of one's experience.

This book is for you. Play with the tracking charts. Have at it. Make your own gorgeous repository and start the exploration. You can begin using the tracking forms at any time that feels right to you. Move through the book as you are tracking based on your own needs.

At the end of your cycle, all you'll need to do is look at the charts you've created. You'll be able to see how hormones and life intertwine. The information is here, ready for you. All you need to do is look and see it. All you need to do is grab a pen.

3.

Tracking Defined

Cycle tracking is the practice of observing the sensations you're feeling, recording them in an organized way, and using that information to learn about yourself and your body's patterns. It's a mindful practice of paying attention to the signs your body and mind are sending to you. It's a practice that can encourage a relationship of trust with your body. It's a process of beginning to listen to your body, feelings, and thoughts and understand how they form the building blocks for every part of your life.

Because many of us have not been given the tools to be present with our bodies, it may feel tough, opaque, and even boring to pay attention to the body's signals. But that doesn't mean it's not possible, achievable, and even pleasurable. We will provide support and guidance every step along the way. We are here in the words, in the guided exercises, and in the charts that are created just for you. We believe in you. You are not alone in this—we are here together. We are here to take good care of you.

While you might be coming to this book because something doesn't feel right, our hope is that you will come to use this method of tracking all the time—when things feel great, when things are humming along, or when things feel hard. When we say tracking for *everyone*, we mean you at any point in your life, no matter what you have going on.

Our bodies are not a static experience. This is why apps often don't work—our bodies are not based on an algorithm. Every chart can be tailored to your needs, and you will be given the tools to engage with your body in the ways that feel best for you based on exactly where you are at that moment in time.

TRACKING FOR SELF-ADVOCACY

The information you gather while tracking will also help you cope with a medical industry that doesn't always welcome self-advocacy. Our current paradigm grapples with a history of systematized discrimination and dismissal of people's medical concerns—especially those of women, LGBTQ+ people, and BIPOC communities. It's common to encounter providers who don't know about cycle tracking or don't ask about the tools their patients use to gain self-knowledge. With a worldwide lack of providers per capita, most medical systems are taxed and unable to direct resources to preventive and chronic care.

These challenges create conditions in which providers might not have the tools to take your concerns seriously. Given limitations around comprehensive assessment, lack of time, and implicit bias—particularly with ethnicity, race, gender, socioeconomic status, and body size—many conditions are misdiagnosed or go undiagnosed, which can leave some people to diagnose themselves.

In her book *In Vitro*, poet Isabel Zapata endures years of narrowly focused medical support while struggling with infertility, wondering why her doctor wasn't taking the health of her partner into consideration. She speaks to the often impossible task of speaking up in a medical setting: "Teetering on the edge of burnout, I often wanted to tell the doctor to seek the problem elsewhere, but I never said a word. It's a silence that still haunts me today. I was paralyzed by the thought of contradicting him."

Even though you have taken the time to observe, collect, and communicate your vital data, the person on the receiving end might not treat it with the gravity it deserves. Self-advocacy can involve an extraordinary amount of emotional labor. We see the time and mental energy that goes into tracking, sharing your data with others, and collaborating in your healthcare planning.

A FEW VERY NORMAL BARRIERS TO TRACKING

Hesitation around tracking is often an understandable result of incomplete sex education, a medical system rife with implicit bias, and a society still struggling with misogyny. It's common to feel aligned with the idea of tracking but a bit averse to *doing* it.

Anxiety and Fear

It may feel scary to imagine what's on the other side of tracking. Protecting ourselves from what we worry might be a difficult diagnosis or an undesirable outcome requiring our time and energy might look like avoiding tracking altogether.

When we see people dig in their heels, we get it. If you feel any of that, it makes sense. We're going to take small steps toward connecting to the body because we know these manageable steps can make a big difference in your overall wellbeing and connection to support. We're going to be right by your side as you make these moves while working with your fear.

Hyperfocus and Compulsivity

For many people, the instruction to pay close attention to regular sensations happening in the body can turn into a cycle of hypervigilance and fixation. A wellmeaning effort to track the body becomes a practice of intense personal focus and sensory overload. The need to tune in may even start to feel compulsive—that is, if you don't track, notice, or analyze every sensation you observe, something "bad" might happen. If you find that your experience ends up feeling more like pressure, we will help you simplify and slow things down.

Overwhelm

Some people just feel completely overwhelmed at the idea of tracking and charts and data. This makes sense! You've got other things to do! However, even with complex, detailed tracking, it can take fewer than five minutes of your day, and tracking even just one or two things can open the door to huge insights.

It's common for our clients to say, "Where do I even begin?" and it's satisfying to share that the answer is so accessible. Tracking can start with the simplest idea. Don't worry, we'll talk you through it on page 38.

Stigma

The moment we start talking about biomarkers like body fluids, plenty of people say, "That's honestly kind of foul, not for me, thank you!" Our culture is squeamish about menstruation and our own anatomy. People don't speak openly about plenty of common bodily experiences. Our aim is to find ways to coexist with our bodies in all their functions. No matter how you might find comfort with your experience of menstruation—and we will guide you through this—you don't have to carry the weight of its historical judgment with you if you don't want to.

Trauma

If you've had a traumatic experience, it's especially crucial to approach the body in a thoughtful way. We've integrated trauma-focused modalities to create a safe and effective way to track. For a more direct guide, see chapter 7, "Dissociation."

A SIMPLE PROCESS WITH OUTSIZE RESULTS

In a nutshell, tracking looks like this:

Get present

Listen in

Identify your goal

Record what you find

Hunt for patterns

Build support

We will help you identify three key pieces of the equation:

Biomarkers

What's going on inside your body

What's happening outside your body

What you will walk away with is invaluable—the ability to tap into your body and track its cycles whenever you want to learn something about yourself. In the future, when something shifts (as it will; our bodies change), imagine feeling prepared instead of startled, able to observe and be comfortable noticing what's happening. When your own needs change (that will happen, too), imagine feeling connected and aware, rather than as if you are starting to get to know your body from scratch.

We do not describe treatments or provide medical advice. That's because we know that nailing this process first is a huge part of getting to the appropriate course of medical action. We are just two people with our own set of lived experiences, and you know best what support looks like for *you*. This book is a vault of personal information about and for you. You can then take it forward. You can decide how to best use the information gleaned.

What comes next is your story to tell.

REAL-LIFE TRACKING

The reasons people come to cycle tracking are, on the surface, diverse. However, hidden in their goals we often discover a universally similar longing—to feel a sense of understanding with their bodies. These stories represent the people we see in our offices, who challenge themselves to follow the process: to explore through journal exercises, record body cues through the charts, and investigate their findings in retrospective reflection. And as a result, they end up with a deeper understanding of themselves.

Nasreen

Nasreen, an elementary school teacher, has wanted children of her own for as long as she can remember. Her friends and family are always impressed by her patience in successfully wrangling a gaggle of kids every day. Her natural optimism and energy have led her to a fulfilling career and have gotten her far in her journey to becoming a parent. However, Nasreen has been trying to conceive for over two years and she notices that her optimism has begun to wane and she doesn't feel like herself. In fact, Nasreen is feeling discouraged, angry, and hopeless.

In a last-ditch effort before starting expensive fertility treatments, Nasreen decides to track. She begins with her biomarkers—her body fluids and basal body temperature—and is going to track results from an ovulation predictor kit, something her doctor had mentioned. Nasreen sets aside five minutes every day to record her results and charges herself with doing this for three cycles.

As Nasreen charts, she looks for ovulation cues, but doesn't notice any during her cycle.

Ines

Ines knows that something doesn't feel right with her body. She has a ton of bloating and pressure in her abdomen before her periods and can't even wear her regular clothes because it is so uncomfortable when her body feels this way.

She has been to twelve different doctors over seven years with no resolution or clarity. Ines performs different versions of what she hopes reads as the "perfect patient" to try to convince these doctors to see and hear her pain. Sometimes she brings all her medical documents and personal research. Other times, she worries that showing up with all of that only ends with the unproductive label of "difficult patient" in her chart. So, on these occasions, she simplifies her woes in a bid to be heard and taken seriously.

Either way, she leaves each appointment without answers. Ironically, Ines works as a patient advocate in a hospital. Ines imagined this would help her navigate the healthcare system, but instead, she feels an additional layer of shame that she hasn't been able to get the support she needs.

Her pain and discomfort impact nearly every part of her life. Ines decides to start tracking to help articulate how this pain manifests. At first, it feels like a slog on top of everything else she has to manage. However, tracking quickly helps provide a cogent picture of everything she has been feeling. Ines is able to express her symptoms in a way that feels accurate to her.

Ines keeps tracking and is determined to get some answers. Ines has an appointment she's been waiting for with a specialist and shares the tracking data she has collected so far. Ines walks out of this appointment with a new diagnosis: endometriosis. Ines continues tracking as she navigates the new world around this diagnosis, and she is also working on rebuilding the trust she has in herself after her experience led her to question her own knowledge of her body.

Ramona

Ramona is a mixed-media artist who is recovering from a bicycle accident. She has been holed up at home resting her knee injury, unable to commute to her studio. She stopped making art and has fallen into a depression.

Forced into stillness, Ramona has to confront changing levels of productivity. As she heals and leans toward creating again, she is struggling with having "off" days. She judges herself for this shift. After a particularly rough week of self-criticism, she knows something needs to change.

Ramona decides to start tracking to help understand some of these hard feelings. She is tracking her biomarkers—body fluids and basal body temperature—and the "on" and "off" days in her studio. So far, tracking is showing her that she tends to have bursts of high creativity around her ovulatory phase and less energy in her luteal phase.

Mei

Mei is in her midtwenties and has been on the hormonal birth control pill for five years. Like most of her friends, she started the pill in high school. Mei has been shown a lot of content on social media about the pill's side effects and is curious about stopping it. The content that resonated the most for Mei was about low mood and change in sexual desire in people on the pill. Mei has been feeling like she is not as excited or close in her relationship as she had once been and is wondering if there might be a hormonal connection.

Mei decides to go off birth control to see what her cycle is like without outside hormones in the picture. Preventing pregnancy is still her primary concern, but she has also heard stories about people experiencing changes in their skin. She wants to be on top of it all.

Mei tries tracking one cycle on an app but is annoyed by the app's hot pink celebratory announcement of her "fertile window." Mei switches to paper and is tracking her mood, skin, sexuality, and ovulation as she transitions off the pill. Mei charts for six cycles as she watches shifts in her body and mood. She wants to know—without any misinformation!—what her options for birth control are.

Sam

Sam, clear about their long-term struggle with body image, comes to cycle tracking looking for support. Sam has gone through periods of dieting, restricting their caloric intake, and desperately trying to change the shape and size of their body since their early teenage years.

The concept of body neutrality really resonates with Sam. Instead of feeling forced to feel amazing about our body if we don't, or the opposite— feeling critical if our body is causing additional pain or distress—a neutral ground can be found through this lens. Replacing a thought like "My body is too big, my lips are too thin, my body is too lazy" with the thought "My body is my home, my body deserves respect" can make a big difference in how we feel. Rather than evaluate through appearance or productivity, the perspective shifts to recognition of function and existence.

Sam is planning to track for three cycles with a goal of body neutrality, and as a first step, they start to track times they feel respect for their body. Sam notices it begins to get easier to feel that respect. It feels like a relief, as if a burden has been lifted off their shoulders. Sam, a triathlete and entrepreneur, loves a challenge and adds pleasure to their daily tracking. The feeling of pleasure that they record is not how they feel about their body but instead when they feel good.

Georgia

Georgia, parent to three children under age six, has been frustrated with the medication she has been prescribed for attention-deficit/hyperactivity disorder (ADHD) for a few years. Sometimes Georgia feels that her medication is working perfectly, and other times she feels so disoriented and off track that she is convinced she needs a new prescription.

Georgia had started tracking her hormonal shifts during pregnancy, postpartum, and nursing. Georgia was not using contraceptives and was diligent about her five minutes of daily tracking. Her cycle had been feeling steady and followed a similar thirtyish-day pattern since the birth of her last child two years before.

At the end of a difficult day with the kids, when she felt her ADHD symptoms were hard to manage, she added two tracking categories related to her focus and concentration. Georgia is tracking these categories for three cycles to learn more about her ADHD.

Talia

Talia feels exasperated when she leaves her meeting. She has been going to a sexual assault support group for a few years and has always found the experience encouraging and validating. Recently, however, Talia has felt distance from her beloved group members and even herself.

On the subway ride home, Talia starts to wonder about what might be contributing to some of these feelings of disconnect. She starts to list things that have changed recently. She is dating someone new and it has been going great. She is proud of the exciting intimate connection she has with her new girlfriend, especially after all the work she had done to feel good in relationships after her childhood sexual trauma.

From her time in her support group, Talia knows a lot about how the body protects itself from traumatic experiences through a feeling of physical disconnect. She has navigated this herself in past romantic relationships and when she was seeing several providers about pelvic pain and pain with sex. In moments when someone else was paying attention to her body, Talia would notice that she felt numb or that she felt as if she were watching herself from the outside.

Talia is curious if her new relationship might be linked to some of these frustrating feelings of disconnect. She already tracks her cycle to help articulate her pain, and she now adds two categories related to disconnection and one related to safety.

As Talia is tracking, she notices a pattern. She begins to suspect that this is not a hormonally connected pattern.

Aisha

For a while, Aisha was convinced that she was going to lose her job. This week has been better at work and what had felt so frightening and overwhelming seems less so. Aisha finds herself breathing a sigh of relief that she no longer believes her job is in jeopardy, but then she feels some anguish when she acknowledges just how hard the previous week had still been. She hadn't been able to sleep more than a few hours each night, was waking up in a pool of sweat in the early morning, felt jittery and restless during the day, and had hardly any appetite. She was short with her family and didn't feel like herself in her relationships.

Aisha thinks back a few cycles to the time when she felt compelled to schedule additional check-ins with her boss. She had been having such *a hard time managing her anxiety about her job security that she needed reassurance. Her boss had seemed perplexed by the third meeting, so Aisha gritted her teeth and made it through the rest of the week. But now, that sense of urgency has seemed to fade away. Aisha had heard a friend talk about how tearful and sad she can feel during certain times of her cycle, and Aisha decides to track hers.*

Aisha notices some changes in her cycle in general. She notes times when she has spiky anxiety, most often about her job security, and she also sees much bigger gaps between bleeding phases.

TRACKING PREP

The basics

The interactive mindfulness exercises woven throughout this book allow us to walk with you as you select the thoughts, emotions, and physical feelings that you will track.

Observing and tracking sensations involves an implicit ask—to pay attention to the body. Non-judgment, openness, and curiosity are powerful tools in this practice. Here there is no pressure to track for anyone else and no pressure to be productive.

You can pick up this book no matter where you find yourself in your day or in your life. These exercises and charts are designed to meet you where you are and can be adapted to your changing needs. Noticing the body's patterns can take a bit of getting used to. On the following pages, we've outlined a quick way to orient yourself to your body. Use this as frequently as you'd like to get connected to your body's signals.

1. SET THE SCENE

Find a space with physical comfort, privacy, and reasonably minimal distraction.

2. GET COMFORTABLE

Find an agreeable position to hang out in. You can be anywhere that feels available. If you'd like, grab pillows and a blanket, or open a window for a gentle breeze—whatever suits your mood.

3. GET PRESENT

Start with a five-minute body scan as an easy and effective way to connect with what's happening inside.

THE BODY SCAN

Observe and bring your attention briefly to each body part.
Practice noticing—starting with your toes and working your
way up to the crown of your head.

BILATERAL PATTERN

If it feels right, you can use a bilateral approach, meaning you
move your attention from one side of the body to the other.
Notice the big toe of your right foot, the big toe of your left
foot, and so on. This can assist with wandering thoughts.

SENSATION OBSERVATION

Notice any sensations at all: tingling, temperature, pressure,
cramping, relaxation, looseness, tightness, buzzing,
fluttering, grinding, numbness . . .

4.

Interconnected Self

As much as the world wants to compartmentalize and organize to better under-stand our existence, our body's complexity will always protest this oversimplifi-cation. Our mental, emotional, physical, and sexual systems are all interrelated. The mental and emotional impacts of how we live in the world are connected to our physical health. Our physical experiences and their impact are connected to our mental and emotional health. In this way, countless studies have shown that what happens inside our bodies affects how we interact with the world outside our bodies, and vice versa. We don't live in a vacuum.

If behavior, environment, biology, and mental well-being are connected, then paying attention to one thing can help you learn about another. The hormonal shifts that come with your cycle can give you a powerful point of entry to taking your body seriously, listening to what it has to tell you, and understanding it in a more thorough way. Listening to the body brings balance and can "accidentally" act as preventive healthcare. Being able to predict discomfort can provide you an opportunity to schedule or seek out support or pleasure.

TRACKING PREP

How to mindfully listen to the body

First, settle into your body. Allow your breathing to calm and slow down a bit. Try to notice what is around you—the things we normally don't pay very much attention to. When you're looking around the space you're in, notice the things you typically wouldn't—for example, the colors of the table in front of you or the movement of a fan. Spend a moment observing the space around you, asking yourself to do nothing more than notice.

Lower your gaze or close your eyes. Turn that observational awareness inward to your body and mind. What do you notice?

When I start paying attention to my senses, a feeling I notice is:

ACTIVE MIND

It is right about now that most people notice just
how very active their mind is and how easy
it is to be distracted. This is natural.

WANDERING THOUGHTS

A thought that is taking my attention away from noticing my body in this moment is:

NON-JUDGMENT

As you notice your thoughts wandering, attempt to
create a vibe free of judgment. Instead of creating a story
about these wandering thoughts, aim for neutrality.
It's not good; it's not bad; it just is.

A critical thought I had about my difficulty staying present is:

A neutral, non-judgmental reframe for my thought is:

HOW DOES MY BODY LOOK?

Don't be surprised if some of the first thoughts
you have when paying attention to your body
are about size, shape, and appearance. This
makes sense when we consider our context:
we live in a world where selling bodies we don't
have is an industry worth hundreds of billions.
When this happens, practice non-judgment and
let the thought pass by. Give yourself permission
to release these thoughts if they come up.

BODY NEUTRALITY

If the experience of judgment around your body
is feeling challenging, consider the framework
of body neutrality. Imagine zero pressure to feel any
which way about your body. You don't have to feel
great and you don't have to feel terrible. Your body
is your home; it doesn't have to define you.
Your body is more than how it looks.
Your body deserves respect.

One thing my body does for me that has nothing to do with appearance is:

THE PRESENT MOMENT

Return to noticing your body. As distracting thoughts
come back, practice: notice them, observe them
without judgment, and allow them to pass by
without engaging. Their content isn't important
right now. You can release them.

Imagine your mind as a vast blue sky; the horizon extends
as far as your mind's eye can see in all directions.
Now, picture each distracting thought as a cloud that
pops up, then dissipates into the vast blue.

*I can picture the clouds in my mind. If I were to draw them, my distracting thought
clouds would look like:*

SELF-COMPASSION

Have compassion for yourself as you work to return your attention back to your body. You are doing something challenging that requires effort and you are doing this because you matter. Imagine your compassion as a color and temperature and visualize it spreading all the way through your entire body, beginning at the crown of your head and moving all the way through, until it reaches your toes.

My self-compassion is the color:

My self-compassion feels like the temperature:

ANCHOR YOUR ATTENTION

We suggest finding an anchor in your body
to focus on when working with wandering thoughts.
For many people, noticing their rhythmic, comforting breath
is an effective anchoring sensation. You might feel your breath
in the expansion and contraction of your lungs, in the rise and fall of
your belly, or in the warmth and gentle sensation of the breath leaving your
nostrils and reaching your upper lip. When your thoughts wander, notice them
with non-judgment, allow them to pass, and return your attention to your breath.

Choose whatever physical anchor works for you.

I look to this part of my body to help anchor me when my attention is wandering:

WHAT CAN YOU TRACK?

Your cycle is about so much more than menstruation. Anything you notice—no matter how big or small—is valid and worth tracking. You can track no matter what hormonal moment you are in. Perhaps you just started menstruating or you are in perimenopause. Tracking is supportive in any stage.

There's no pressure to capture every single bodily cue. Nor is there a particular pace at which you should track. If you miss a few days of logging, the information you've gathered is still useful. Track at a pace that works best for you.

If you have a chronic condition, tracking can be particularly helpful. We often see clients coping with chronic autoimmune concerns. In fact, most people with autoimmune conditions, around 80 percent, are people assigned female at birth. Hormonal shifts can change the way symptoms of chronic health struggles are expressed and felt. Because these conditions can impact every part of how your body feels, these cues can help you understand your experience.

We're going to take you through different cues, including prompts to investigate your own sensations. You'll notice a mix of descriptive, feelings-based prompts as well as more clinical, symptom-based prompts. The beauty of a wide spectrum of sensations is that we can all find a place on it. For both of us and our clients, the biggest aha moment can be realizing we had assumed a tracking sensation had a particular "good" or "bad" value. Consider the categories you choose to track from a neutral lens; they are neither right nor wrong, and you determine your priorities over time. These are starting points for your exploration, here to serve as a way into reflection about what might be relevant for you.

Body Cues

Every cycle tells a story. Tracking your menstrual patterns can help providers identify health concerns. For instance, cycle variability can aid in diagnosing conditions such as polycystic ovary syndrome (PCOS, also known as metabolic reproductive syndrome) and thyroid disease. But it's not only critical for clinicians and providers to understand your cycle, it's also essential for *you* to understand it, to find *your* normal, and to give yourself tools to advocate for yourself to those providers when something feels off. While you might be aware of the bodily cues you feel regularly, this is an invitation to expand into less familiar areas.

BODY CUES TO CONSIDER

- **Body fluids**
  - Color
  - Amount
  - Odor
  - Texture
  - Quality

- **Digestion**
  - Constipation or diarrhea
  - Increase or decrease in appetite or satiation
  - Shift in blood sugar and hunger cues
  - Aversions or nausea
  - Pressure or cramping

- **Energy**
  - Fatigue or alertness
  - Clarity or fuzziness
  - Fiery or cool
  - Sleep is available or disrupted
  - Dreams are vivid or fleeting

- **Sensory**
  - Overload or not enough
  - "Touched out" or craving physical soothing
  - Hyperfocused or generalized
  - *Yes* to stimulation or in need of a break and a reset

- **Body tissues (skin, hair, nails . . .)**
  - ▸ Oily or dry
  - ▸ Brittle or strong
  - ▸ Thinning or thickening
  - ▸ Presence or absence of common skin changes
    - › For example: acne, eczema, herpes 1 and 2, psoriasis, dandruff

- **Pleasure**
  - ▸ Feeling good through touch
  - ▸ Peace in your body
  - ▸ Joy, happiness, or elation in self and connection
  - ▸ Delight in the senses
  - ▸ Catharsis through movement

- **Pain**
  - ▸ Tension or cramping
  - ▸ Throbbing or aching
  - ▸ Heaviness or pressure
  - ▸ Itching or burning
  - ▸ Stabbing or punching

- **Chronic**
  - ▸ Presence or absence of health symptoms
  - ▸ Intensity of chronic sensations
  - ▸ Emotions about health feeling heavy or light
  - ▸ Feeling present or distracted in life

Emotional Cues

Hormonal shifts can have a powerful impact on mood, mental health, and emotionality, creating a potentially wide spectrum of feelings and thoughts. There's no denying the correlations between hormone fluctuation and symptoms of mental health experiences such as depression, anxiety, obsessive-compulsive disorder (OCD), post-traumatic stress disorder (PTSD), and borderline person-ality disorder. Studies demonstrate a shift in many symptoms at various cyclical moments.

The connection is right there. Because the physical and the mental are inex-tricably linked, changes to emotional health can also affect feelings within the body, impacting your whole being as you move through your cycle.

EMOTIONAL CUES TO CONSIDER

- **Feelings within the body**
  - ▸ Lightness or heaviness
  - ▸ Tension or tightness
  - ▸ Pressure or constriction
  - ▸ Soreness or softness
  - ▸ Buzzing or tingling
  - ▸ Breathing or heart rate changes
  - ▸ Sweating or dryness
  - ▸ Loose or controlled

- **Feelings of anxiety and depression**
  - ▸ Fixations and obsessions
  - ▸ Hopelessness
  - ▸ Pervasive worry
  - ▸ Excessive anger toward self or others
  - ▸ Panic and fear

- **Feelings about yourself and the world around you**
  - ▸ Confidence
  - ▸ Self-criticism
  - ▸ Empowerment
  - ▸ Reactionary

- **Feelings with other people**
  - Connected or disconnected
  - Increased irritation or adoration
  - Desire for intimacy or independence
  - Loneliness and isolation

- **Feelings about reality and connection to self**
  - Paranoia and fear
  - Feeling that you have new and extraordinary abilities
  - Worry that others are out to get you
  - Time passing without realizing it
  - Major disruptions in maintaining regular schedule

Cognitive Cues

The concept of the "embodied brain" underscores the way our physical selves relate to our cognitive processes and the inseparable relationship between the two. They both reside in the body, making them similarly connected to our physical well-being.

Whether you identify as neurodivergent, identify as a person with ADHD or OCD, or notice variability in your cognition, you'll find that tracking is an invaluable exploration. Once you have a baseline for your body and mind, you're better equipped to identify when something doesn't feel right. Understanding your cycle's impact on your cognitive functions is all about figuring out what your norm looks like.

COGNITIVE CUES TO CONSIDER

- **Awareness**
  - Alertness or fatigue
  - Foggy or precise
  - Clear or jumbled

- **Creativity**
  - Stimulated or stifled
  - Free-flowing or stuck
  - Abundant or dry

- **Motivation**
  - Energized or unmotivated
  - Lightness or heaviness
  - Moving or stopped

- **Attention**
  - Focused or blurry
  - Disjointed or fine-tuned
  - Short or prolonged
  - Everywhere or one place

- **Integration**
  - Feeling like yourself
  - Ability to engage in your activities of importance
  - Energy to connect with others

- **Rest**
  - Accessible or challenging
  - Racing thoughts or calm
  - Regular or disrupted

- **Culture**
  - Engagement with music
  - Response to art
  - Relationship to personal expression, appearance
  - Intensity of feeling about political moments

Sexual Cues

Feeling shifts in sexual desire is normal!

Understanding the ways your cycle impacts your sexuality can be clarifying and can help you communicate your needs to yourself and your partner(s) or advocate for what feels best. Many of us have been socialized by external cultural ideals of what sex is supposed to look like, which build powerful narratives around what is "healthy" and what is not, what we should or shouldn't want sexually, and which feelings or acts are "right" and which are "wrong." Sexuality, arousal, and desire exist on a vast spectrum, rather than a narrow assumption of normalcy.

Hormonal shifts can have a big influence on sexuality. When tracking, it may be tempting to use the markers for sexuality we often see reflected around us, like frequency and type of sex. But these two criteria come up woefully short when describing sexuality for our clients. Instead of prioritizing the amount and type of sex that one is having, we see in our work that it is much more enlightening to explore the distinct sensations of a person's own sexual and erotic self, knowing that this is flexible and can even look different day to day, moment to moment.

In their book *Refusing Compulsory Sexuality*, Sherronda J. Brown writes about the societal pressure to perform a certain amount and kind of sexuality. "Compulsory sexuality allows for a tacit refusal or inability to accept the idea that we all have the inherent right to govern our own bodies and make our own decisions about whether or not to engage in sex, and that we can do this based on whatever criteria we deem fit." Brown goes on to explain, "Narrow ideas of sexuality can also work to obscure and diminish the nonnormative ways that erotic lives can manifest themselves."

When tracking sexual cues, we encourage casting a wide net to capture all of the ways you may experience this part of yourself, not just the typical application of sexuality, which may not feel like the right fit anyway. For some, romance is connected to sexuality; for others, it is not. The same goes for sexual attraction—for some, sexual attraction is a part of their sexuality; for others, it is not. Sexuality is not dependent on another person, and many of these prompts are about only you.

Studies have found that progesterone—the regulating hormone—tends to decrease sexual arousal, while estrogens tend to increase it. You may notice cycle patterns that seem to reliably follow this hormonal shift: perhaps a lift in erotic feelings toward the middle of your cycle, when estrogens peak, and a dip when they decrease. These trends aren't true for every person, nor do they manifest in the same way for every body.

Listen to your cues throughout your cycle and determine what matters most to you.

SEXUAL AND EROTIC CUES TO CONSIDER

- **Closeness and intimacy**
  - ▸ Feeling openness or protection toward connection
  - ▸ Desire for reliability or interest in new, adventurous erotic expression
  - ▸ Readiness for touch from another person or outside touch feels intrusive

- **Pleasure and discomfort**
  - ▸ Presence or absence of physical or emotional pain or discomfort with sexual touch
  - ▸ Intensity of pleasure or enjoyment with erotic touch
  - ▸ Feeling affirmed or disconnected in your body
  - ▸ Changes in your response to your partner's body or partners' bodies
  - ▸ Changes in lubrication

- **Arousal and desire**
  - ▸ Physical and emotional response to sexual touch and erotic connection
  - ▸ Presence or absence of sexual, erotic thoughts
  - ▸ Feeling "turned on" or "turned off"
  - ▸ Change in context and length of time related to arousal or orgasm

- **Sexuality and connection**
  - Shifting emotional and sexual dynamics with others
  - Changes in power balance with others
  - Changes in sensory experiences like touch and smell when connecting with partner(s)
  - "Turned on" by or drawn to new or different people, imagery, objects of interest, or activities
  - Shifts in romantic interest or feelings

Relationship Cues

Fluctuations of connectedness in your personal relationships—relationships of every type—are to be expected. When these fluctuations feel foreign or uncomfortable, you may find that exploring these changes in the context of cyclical hormones is helpful.

Hormonal shifts may correspond with varying levels of ease in communication and levels of comfort in physical and emotional closeness.

RELATIONSHIP CUES TO CONSIDER

- **Communication styles**
  - Direct or indirect language
  - Shortness or patience with listening
  - Calm or aggressive tones
  - Neutral or defensive responses

- **Energetic needs**
  - Extroverted or introverted
  - Self-regulation through closeness or regulation through alone time
  - Stillness or restlessness with others

- **Proximity comfort**
  - ▸ Shifting feelings of isolation and loneliness
  - ▸ Changes in ease of connection with others
  - ▸ Feeling more or less social

- **Meaning and community connection**
  - ▸ Shift with personal spirituality, religion, or higher power
  - ▸ Existential grounding or discomfort
  - ▸ Different awareness of sense of purpose
  - ▸ Community closeness or disengagement
  - ▸ Changing relationship to superstition

TRACKING PREP

You and the systems around you

The idea that our individual lifestyle changes and choices have the greatest impact on our bodies is a misconception: research shows that about 65 percent of health outcomes are based on other factors including socioeconomics, our environment, and the clinical care system we do (or don't) have access to.

These social determinants of health are a piece of the puzzle.

We all live in a series of intersecting systems. Some are shared, but many are particular to us as individuals. These systems can have an enormous impact on our options and, ultimately, on our lives.

VISUALIZE YOURSELF WITHIN

THE SYSTEMS AROUND YOU

How has your life been impacted by the systems around you?

Do any of these systemic experiences feel connected to you or your life? If so, draw a line connecting yourself (ME) to the different micro and macro systems around you. Write anything about these systems that relates to you personally.

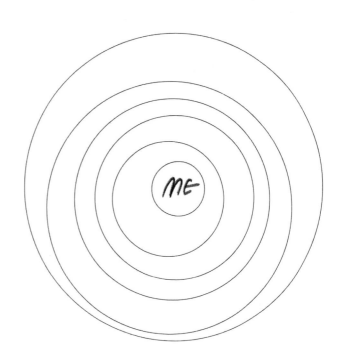

SOCIAL STRUCTURE

CAREGIVERS

EDUCATION

NEIGHBORHOOD

SEXUALITY

FAMILY

MEDIA

FRIENDS

SOCIOECONOMICS

GENDER

SCHOOL

SPIRITUALITY

MONEY

CULTURE

MEDICAL

RELIGION

GEOGRAPHY

My life has been particularly impacted by these systems:

I feel supported by these systems:

I feel limited by these systems:

The feeling I have in my body when I think about how these systems have shaped my life is:

5.

Pleasure

The foundation of this book is built on a specific experience of pleasure—the pleasure that comes from the practice of listening to the body. There is pleasure in trusting your instincts and in finding freedom through a relationship with the body defined by you and you alone.

What's more, if you start tracking pleasure, you're going to start feeling pleasure.

Consumer culture defines pleasure narrowly: bubble baths and "self-care," rom-coms and soft, languorous kisses. There are some people who would have you believe that only certain expressions of pleasure are acceptable. Ignore them. We encourage a deep dive inward to explore a personal connection to the sensorial *feelings* of pleasure. What are those tiny individual moments in which you feel really good?

Tracking those moments can be transformative.

What does this pleasure feel like for you? Where does it show up? How is it held in your body?

You may define pleasure as a spectrum of individualized sensations like satisfaction, joy, delight, euphoria, or bliss. You may experience sympathetic pleasure from making someone else feel good. Pleasure can be responsive or spontaneous. Pleasure may come as a result of something that doesn't feel good in the process, like hard work, and you may derive pleasure from certain types of pain.

THE PAIN-PLEASURE SPECTRUM

*Pleasure for me, doesn't exclude or deny pain. The same self, the same
inclusive awareness that allows me to experience pleasure, may retreat
or cramp up in the face of pain (physical or emotional) but returns,
and so far, is always bigger and able to absorb or metabolize it.*

—ALTA STARR, QUOTED IN *PLEASURE ACTIVISM: THE POLITICS OF FEELING GOOD*

Pain and pleasure are often depicted in opposition.

Seeing things as binary and mutually exclusive is understandable. It is easier, more palatable, to take in two individual options rather than a big, gray, overlapping spectrum. While many people experience pleasure separate from pain, as those with chronic illness or pain are acutely aware, pleasure may also coexist with ever-present pain.

When you are investigating pain, pleasure may feel completely absent. In fact, if you're tracking something difficult or painful, we recommend that you also track pleasure. In *Pleasure Activism*, a collection of interviews by writer and activist adrienne maree brown, brown speaks to Alana Devich Cyril, living at the time with late-stage cancer. Cyril shared, "I believe in pleasure as a practice. You can fall out of practice, but life is so much better when you're exercising your pleasure muscles."

A type of pleasure that we love to work with we call *comfort*. Comfort encompasses feelings of safety and ease.

Nasreen

*As Nasreen explores her desire to have children and her subsequent
treatment options, she copes with feelings of hypervigilance and the feeling
that she must constantly take action. Comfort means peace and rest as she
works with infertility. Nasreen finds that for her, comfort represents the other
side of that stress spectrum.*

Ines

Ines has been dealing with distracting cycle pain for so long now. For Ines, comfort is a physical feeling of calm and power. The feeling is distinct and she has noticed it more throughout her quest to get answers and support for her pain.

Ramona

As Ramona explores the ebbs and flows of creativity and productivity in her art practice, she identifies comfort as an understanding of her body's patterns. The more she feels connected, the more often she notices comfort in her life. She finds ease in knowing that times that feel tough won't last forever.

Mei

Mei has been adjusting to how her body feels off birth control. At first comfort was hard to identify, but Mei realizes that for her, comfort is the feeling that she can trust herself and her body. She learns that she doesn't need to be so concerned about herself and can listen to her body without pressure to "fix" or "solve."

Sam

At first Sam thought their struggles with body image meant they weren't able to find comfort in their life. But for Sam, comfort is a stable, easy feeling. It is often the absence of a feeling of conflict with their body, and sometimes Sam notices comfort when they realize that it's been a while since they had a self-critical thought.

Georgia

Georgia's feeling of comfort is specific to where she is in life right now. Comfort is a newer feeling. Georgia comes into a recently discovered version of herself after weaning her third child. Comfort means a sense of calm within her body and a connection to her identity.

Talia

As Talia has been exploring her relationship with her girlfriend, she finds that her feeling of comfort is currently connected to her attachment and relationships. Comfort means safety and trust within her relationships. This feeling is a restful reassurance.

Aisha

When Aisha starts to look at what makes anxiety days feel different than quiet days at work, she can see that for her, comfort is about her personal agency. When Aisha feels access to her own internal choices and options, she feels strong, well-resourced, and peaceful.

Discovering even a tiny amount of pleasure in a cycle can also be a useful tool to better understand how to manage pain. For example, approaching a cyclical point of pain with a planned balance of pleasure might mitigate your overall discomfort. By taking a wide poll of your sensations, you gain perspective. The broader the spectrum of sensations you track, the better your data set is to analyze and understand yourself.

THE PLEASURE OF TRACKING

We don't always give ourselves credit for doing difficult things.

You may find that daily tracking is a painful reminder that something doesn't feel the way you think it should. But prioritizing this hard work today can make things easier and better for future you.

Recognizing how hard you're working and how strong and committed you are to supporting your future self is also something that can feel good. That's the pleasure of tracking when you don't want to be tracking.

You are here. To access pleasure in connection to the self while also noticing pain requires a psychological feat—holding space for two seemingly contradictory ideas and feelings at once.

In fact, it's a superpower.

WHEN PLEASURE FEELS COMPLICATED

Pleasure can also be protective.

If you are using this book to track behaviors that don't feel like they are serving you, this might be a useful concept to consider. Seeking activities and experiences that feel good in the face of emotional or physical pain is a useful adaptation. Trying to feel better and attempting to lessen hurt is understandable. No one wants to suffer.

You may find that it feels more natural to notice painful, uncomfortable, or undesirable bodily sensations than attempting to articulate and track pleasurable ones. You are not alone. The gaps in what so many of us have been taught about our bodies not only hinder our understanding of functioning and anatomy, they can also limit our understanding of bodily enjoyment.

TRACKING RECOMMENDATIONS:

1. Start with one easy-to-identify pleasurable sensation. By *easy-to-identify*, we mean something that you can quickly and regularly feel without strenuous efforts. Laughter, relaxation, a sensation of connection—these are all good examples. Find yours, it's different for us all.

2. Add this as a tracking category for one to three cycles.

3. Observe the ways in which this pleasure might feel different through tracking it.

4. Add additional, more complex pleasure tracking categories to your charts as time goes on.

You are amazing. If that feels hard to hear, it might be worth pausing a moment and considering why. We spend a lot of time devaluing ourselves and second-guessing our worth.

You are amazing.

TRACKING PREP

Your body is yours; your pleasure is yours

We absorb messages from a young age about how the world works as we observe the ways people behave around us. We receive information through direct communication and through more subtle body language cues, relationship dynamics, and ways people we know take care of themselves. We see reductive representation in media, music, and politics. There may be topics that were avoided completely in our childhood; we receive that message loud and clear. "Don't talk about it, don't let anyone see, hide it." This is an opportunity ripe for shame—without modeling, without examples, we may fear that who we are is not okay.

You might realize at some point that these internalized beliefs are not working for you. Unlearning messages we absorbed a long time ago can be complicated. In our practices, we look to each person's own story to help.

We like to be curious about past messages and understand why we might have some of the beliefs that we do. Once we've done this investigation, we get to really turn these beliefs over and ask ourselves, "What do I want to do with this thought? Does it serve me? Do I keep it or release it?"

You are full of wisdom and knowledge about what feels right and good for you.

Your body is yours.

You get to decide how you want to listen to it, talk to it, and take care of it.

Let's take a journey back through your memories.
Don't worry about identifying anything exact;
we are here to illuminate connections between
what was modeled to you and what you feel today.
It's also worth noting if you can recall not the presence
of some of these prompts but the absence.

PLEASURE

When I was younger, I saw the essential people in my life feel good when they were:

In my memory, the first time pleasure *was defined for me was:*

An old belief I have about pleasure that no longer serves me is:

I remember understanding what people meant when they were talking about "sex" when:

MEMORIES

Pleasure in your body is felt through the lens of how you've been taught to feel about your body. Consider some of what you learned when you were younger.

I heard the essential people in my life talk about their bodies by saying:

The essential people in my life took care of their bodies by:

A time when someone talked to me about my body in a way that didn't feel good was:

A time when someone talked to me about my body in a way that felt great was:

Ways I like others to talk about my body:

WHEN MY BODY FEELS GOOD

it feels:

- ○ warm
- ○ cozy
- ○ breezy
- ○ light
- ○ flowing
- ○ twinkling
- ○ expanding
- ○ glowing
- ○ soft
- ○ spiky
- ○ tickly
- ○ slinky
- ○ sexy

- ○ squishy
- ○ hazy
- ○ sunny
- ○ electric
- ○ cloudy
- ○ icy
- ○ flickering
- ○ full
- ○ glistening
- ○ rested
- ○ _____
- ○ _____
- ○ _____

6.

Safety

If you've experienced trauma, we are profoundly sorry. That should not have happened. It is not right, just, or fair. You deserve to be taken care of.

Trauma can rob us of our sense of safety, leaving us operating in a protective mode without rest. Because the body and mind have powerful protective systems in place, even identifying trauma might not be possible until safety is broached. If you have decided to investigate trauma in your life, it is crucial to also identify individual systems of safety. Where trauma dysregulates, safety regulates.

Our clients coping with trauma describe feeling uninterested in tracking or engaged in a minimal way because it is not yet safe to be in their bodies. Keeping their distance has been protective. These clients want to learn more so they can feel better but get stuck when trying to use tracking as a method to get there.

You can still track even if you've experienced trauma.

When our clients come into our offices with past trauma, they usually start with a description of what feels unsafe. What *doesn't* feel safe is clear to us all as we sit together in conversation and feel the vibration of that pain and the heaviness of that fear. Sometimes, witnessing a client's post-traumatic response translates into a feeling of pressure, an attempt to solve something, *anything*, for that person. But instead of jumping into problem-solving mode, we've come to realize that the first step toward meaningful resolution for that client is finding personal, unique safety within.

The great thing about working with personal safety is that it can be done at any pace and in conjunction with other paths of healing and medical treatment. We are working toward a feeling of "safe enough," knowing that we do not need to find a sense of *total* safety to feel regulated and calm.

Finding personal safety highlights your strengths and reminds you of your inherent wisdom.

Safety is a sense of security and comfort within yourself. In part, this comes from a confidence that your choices are yours to make. Safety is a feeling of calm and a belief that you don't have to always be on high alert.

Rest is accessible.

Your body is the vessel in which you live. It doesn't have to be who you are.

PERSONAL AGENCY

There is so much you can do by engaging with your body, not just by "fixing" what's "bad" and "broken" but also by uncovering and embracing your ability to self-regulate.

We all have the right to personal determination regarding what happens to our bodies. This right is not always reflected in the systems around us. The relationship between people and structures of power is so fraught that some have attempted to solve this through explicitly detailed contracts defining consent, informed choice, and shared decision-making. While these attempts offer some protection to people within these systems, personal agency involves more than a legal contract.

Bodily agency is a feeling of awareness, choice, and possibility in relationship to yourself and your life. This feeling can be abstract and personal, individualized and specified. You get to turn your attention inward and define this yourself. The existence of your personal agency can provide safety and protection against trauma.

When another person touches, references, or treats your body in a way that you know isn't right, it may dramatically affect the way you exist within yourself. When this happens, you may not have access to self-determination.

The imbalance of people and systems in power can be a contributing factor in the experience of trauma, causing suffering. Social and institutional inequity in the form of body-shaming, coercion, and harassment can lead to the loss of personal agency. With this discrimination, you aren't being seen or taken care of.

The ways that people have mistreated us can color how we view ourselves, damaging the words we use in our minds and the ways we assess our own value. Safety encourages a reconnection to our strength and that feeling of comfort. You get to choose when you want to access this feeling or not. You might choose to use it during times when you know you are safe and yet you don't *feel* safe. What we see in our practices is that actively inviting times of calm and peace can mitigate the impacts of trauma and reduce instances of hypervigilance and fear.

Approaching the body with a sense of care and neutrality can be useful when working to reconnect to a feeling of personal agency. There's no right or wrong way to have a body.

BODY NEUTRALITY

Another way to feel safe is through body neutrality. We are constantly pushed and pulled to feel certain ways about our bodies—from media images that demand we be a certain shape and size, to body positivity movements that encourage us to celebrate and love our bodies, to the medical industry that often shames us for the things we do or don't do with them. People—especially women, BIPOC people, and others from marginalized communities—are often told what they should look like, what sensations they should be experiencing, and what they should feel about their bodies.

Here, there is no *should*.

In our work, we see how good it can feel to center what the body *does*, rather than what it looks like, without judgment or pressure to feel a certain way about it. We want to remove any binary expectations—good/bad, love/hate, cynicism/ optimism—about what connecting with your body looks like.

To engage with your body, you don't need to love or hate it. You don't even have to identify with it. You only need to listen to what it's telling you. Through this approach, you're able to be open and honest with yourself about what your body *is* feeling, rather than what it should be feeling.

Sam

Sam has spent a lot of energy trying to ignore their body. In times when the size and shape of their body doesn't feel right, Sam experiences a sense of panic and overload when getting dressed, looking in the mirror, and when hearing other people talk about their own bodies. Sam finds it difficult not to fixate on the types of bodies and identities they see promoted around them. Their thoughts turn to ways they can "work" to change their body. In some ways, these thoughts feel productive, because Sam can take steps to make their body look different. But with some perspective, they can see that these thoughts are relentless.

On many days, it feels like a reprieve to not feel their body at all. But Sam notices that this disconnect doesn't seem to be making them feel any better, either. It is becoming increasingly hard to take good care of their body. Embracing their body full-on feels overwhelming, so they begin to adopt a body-neutral perspective.

Sam slowly begins to pay attention to their body again, first by recognizing the parts that feel easier to connect with. Sam starts with their feet. As Sam notices how much their body does for them that has nothing to do with appearance or size, they find it possible to respect their body and even to be a bit in awe. Sam practices looking in the mirror and, instead of fixating on their body size, thinking, "My body does so much every day." On days when it feels more difficult to be present in their body without feelings of self-criticism, Sam reminds themself that even though they are at home in their body, it does not define them.

After a few months of shifting the way they think about their body, Sam feels ready to start tracking. They are considering a few birth control options and would like to have a solid understanding of their cycle so they can make an informed choice. Because Sam integrates body-neutral sensations into their tracking, they're afforded even more practice reframing their harsh thoughts.

Coexisting with their body becomes easier and easier until it happens without them realizing it. Sam uses the comfort tracking category to note days when they feel they are in easy dialogue with their body instead of in battle.

These are days they are able to listen to what their body needs and provide it. Sam is able to start participating in their healthcare and is experiencing more and more days in which they appreciate and feel safe in their body.

TAKE CARE OF YOURSELF

Introducing safety tracking into your chart can make the tracking experience feel more sustainable.

When we're working with a new client, we start a dialogue to explore what they want to track. We offer a whole slew of examples to start. We also suggest tracking safety—but instead of saying "tracking safety," we ask, "Is there any particular form of movement you do in your body that feels good to you? How do you like to nourish your body? What kinds of things bring you calm? What brings you energy?"

From their different and always interesting answers, we find some approachable sensations to track. We encourage the inclusion of pleasure, especially when managing pain. We watch a person's connection to personal safety grow through these exercises.

TRACKING RECOMMENDATIONS:

1. It takes time to get used to the experience of noticing comfort, not just discomfort. Give yourself extra patience as you begin tracking sensations that feel good, grounding, and calming.

2. Start by using the safety tracking category of *comfort*, included in every tracking chart. Continue with this until you feel ease and mastery in accessing this sensation. Once you feel like you can notice and engage with that *one* feeling when you want to and when it's helpful, experiment with expanding.

3. Add more safety tracking categories from this point.

4. Making daily choices to reject messages of shame or to claim experiences of pleasure is often a lifelong endeavor. Consider creating a category to recognize and celebrate your efforts.

TRACKING PREP

Finding internal safety

This exercise
uses visualization techniques
to connect with
sensations of safety
to use in times of need.

In a moment of feeling flooded by a trauma response, dissociated, and removed from the body, we can come back into ourselves by calling upon feelings of comfort and grounding bodily sensations.

Recall the last time you felt any of the following:

POWERFUL
STRONG
CALM
PRESENT
AFFIRMED

When was the last time you felt like yourself? *Truly like yourself.*

Go to that place, call upon that moment, and try to envision: What were the colors, temperatures, and sensations?

What comes to mind when I put myself in that place . . .

The COLOR is:

The TEMPERATURE is:

The LANDSCAPE is:

My BODILY SENSATION is:

My EMOTION is:

Now let's turn these abstract sensations into something trackable and concrete (e.g., "The color blue makes me feel at ease").

My *COLOR* makes me feel:

My *TEMPERATURE* makes me feel:

My *LANDSCAPE* makes me feel:

My *BODILY SENSATION* makes me feel:

My *EMOTION* makes me feel:

Here are some commonly felt sensations related to trauma. Are there times you can identify feeling any of them? Write whatever comes to mind.

I feel *TENSE* when:

I feel *NUMB* when:

I feel *UNEASY* when:

I feel *BLAH* when:

I feel *REPULSED* when:

I feel _____ when:

Activating the details of your visualization in a time when
you notice stress, or even a trauma response, acts as a bridge to safety.
Feeling the sensation of warmth on your face is ground gained
toward feeling your body. Feeling your body is a step toward safety
and self-regulation, and away from a trauma response.

my COMFORT FEELS LIKE:

WHAT COMFORT MEANS TO ME:

7.

Dissociation

"I had cleaved myself from my body long ago. This was nothing new."

In her book *Touched Out*, Amanda Montei describes the ways she used dissociation as a coping method. In her memories of adolescence and sexual moments in which she felt silenced, she writes, "Over time, I became conscious that my body did not belong only to me. It was a tapestry to be admired or reviled, a tool to be used, a voice to be silenced, a vessel for reproduction, and a product to be primed for consumption."

So many of us have lived through painful moments in which we did not feel our bodies were treated the way they should have been, did not feel as if what happened to our bodies was in our control, and were silenced. Dissociation is one way to cope.

We believe in the strength of the body and the mind. How incredible is it that we are able to create ways to move forward, even in the face of pain and trauma? The body and the mind forge protective and defensive coping methods in brilliant adaptation.

Years in our practices have informed our approach to working with trauma in the body. It leads to much better outcomes for our clients when we delve into how and why the body and mind created these adaptations, rather than viewing them as pathologies or dysfunctions.

DISSOCIATION AS PROTECTION

Dissociation is the process of disconnecting from ourselves as a protection from discomfort, pain, and suffering. If we aren't present, we might be sheltered from some of the experience. Dissociation exists to allow you a reprieve from trauma. When you are dissociating, your mind is quite literally escaping. This means that when you are dissociating, you are often not aware that it is happening. This is exactly how dissociation is intended to work. We often hear it described by our clients as *numbing*, *void*, *zoning out*, *fuzziness*, and *floating away from my body*. Sometimes people feel as if they are watching themselves from outside their body. You might notice that time has passed without you realizing it.

We regularly see dissociation and have come to find that naming and understanding this experience can help people better understand and regulate themselves. This response shows up in quite a few of our clients, and at first, it often feels like a barrier to tracking. However, once we've identified this adaptive reaction, there are a lot of different, really effective ways we can work with it.

Sex educator and activist Staci Haines highlights five main protective adaptations: fight, flight, freeze, appease, and dissociate.

These adaptations are usually activated automatically and occur without conscious recognition or request. You may not even know that one of these responses has been set off until you find yourself in it.

FIGHT:
DEFEND

FLIGHT:
REDIRECT

As part of these protective responses, the body and mind are on high alert for anything that echoes the previously experienced danger or resembles a burgeoning hazard. This can feel like living in a state of terror or, alternately, when it is simply too much to maintain this level of hypervigilance, a state of numbness. The effects of this can permeate nearly every part of your life and can be expressed in emotions, behavior, sensory experiences, relationships, attachment, cognition, sexuality, and so on.

By uncovering these patterns, we can begin to move forward.

DISSOCIATION AS HABIT

Dissociation is very useful while trauma is happening. It can automatically turn on to save you from that moment, but after a trauma is over, it doesn't always automatically turn off. It can also turn on unexpectedly with just a faint reminder of that trauma.

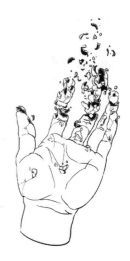

So many of our clients have had to confront sexual violations. Their bodies and minds are often primed to

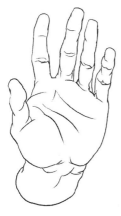

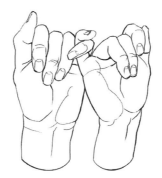

FREEZE:
IMMOBILIZE

APPEASE:
PLACATE

DISSOCIATE:
DISCONNECT

have a protective response to anything that reminds them of those traumas. The body is so ready to go into protective mode that in some instances the whole pelvic region goes offline. It can be hard or frustrating for them to access pleasure or connection in romantic relationships, more so when they really want that intimacy. Even in moments when they intellectually recognize that they are safe, they realize that their body has disconnected. This distancing from the body, the comfort gained in being away from it, can understandably become habitual. The cumulative effect of this can be an overall numbing to the body and its signals.

Trauma

In this moment, when people are being both over- and underdiagnosed with mental health conditions, when *trauma* is both a ubiquitous buzzword and a life-changing reframe, it can be especially confusing to try to understand your own experiences. Trauma is pervasive, and its effects on the body may sneak up on you. It can fundamentally change how it feels to be in our bodies.

In moments of trauma, your body and mind go to extraordinary lengths to try to protect you.

And because trauma is so frequently misidentified, misunderstood, and misrepresented, people often don't even realize the extent to which it has impacted their lives.

We see clients show up because they want to learn more about their bodies so they can feel better, but they feel stuck when trying to use tracking as a method to get there.

There are a lot of reasons why it is hard to treat the symptoms of trauma. A thorough assessment might be required to distinguish exactly how that trauma affects us physically and emotionally, a process that is complicated for both the individual and the provider.

Pressure to be strong, especially mentally and emotionally, is widespread. This internalized expectation leads many of us to have unrealistic ideas of how we should respond to trauma, denying how much it might have impacted us. The stigma around mental and emotional pain is unfortunately alive and well, held deep within many of us.

CAUSES WE ENCOUNTER

We've noticed some themes in our practices around dissociation as they relate to our clients' goals with their bodies. The air we breathe and the violence to our bodies that we've survived contribute to this protective response.

Living in the World

Maybe you're reading this right now and thinking, "That's not my issue." But, if trauma is pervasive, then it only follows that dissociation is, too. The world we live in fosters and encourages dissociation. Technology, false authority, suppressive systems, gender inequity, lack of free access to information—it all separates us from our bodies.

We see a slow and steady erosion of bodily awareness that comes from impossible beauty standards, shame, pressure to perform, and subtle systemic oppression. We are hurt by an accumulation of instances in which our preferences are overridden because of the belief that others' pleasure matters more than our own. We're told repeatedly about the assessed value of our body, and so many of us are trained to evaluate ourselves based on these false standards.

The world we live in has created a disconnect. In many ways, we've been taught not to trust our knowledge of our own bodies. We wonder if we are accurately interpreting what we are feeling—that is, if we've even been granted access to explore those feelings at all.

Body-Based Violence

There are times in which the well-being of your body is in the hands of someone else. We see clients who were harmed when they entrusted their body to someone in a medical setting, or when someone enacted physical or sexual violence on them.

When we work with people who have experienced trauma, we listen carefully to how each individual prefers to talk about and name the parts of their bodies that have been affected. We use that shared language that feels best. Sometimes there isn't a clear way to talk about bodies that feels right, and sometimes it feels better to have someone else come up with the language. When this happens, we have found that using neutral, descriptive terminology makes space for everyone's story.

Please use your own language to describe your body and its parts. If you'd like, exchange the neutral terminology we use—*the pelvis* and *the genitals*—for whatever words work for you.

If your trauma has involved your bodily agency or parts of your body that are directly impacted by your cycle, like your pelvis and genitals, you may run into protective responses like disconnect and numbing as you direct your attention to your body. It may be a sign that your body is overwhelmed by the trauma it has experienced and should be approached with care.

Let's consider what can happen when someone's body is mistreated. Because rape and sexual violence are currently some of the top causes of PTSD, this means a person's body, genitals, and sexuality are often affected. It is common to have levels of dissociation in and around your chest, vulva, vagina, and abdomen, and all the other parts of your body that feel connected to your sexuality, fertility, and cycle.

This person carries with them painful memories associated with their body or certain parts of their body. Enter dissociation—the useful coping method to allow this person to move through life without confronting this memory every time they think of, or feel, their body. Not noticing, or choosing not to feel, these body parts (chest, abdomen, vulva, vagina) can help them feel free of the physical and emotional pain by not feeling at all.

If a memory associated with your genitals involves someone mistreating them, or not taking your pleasure or safety into consideration, or even giving you the message that you are to feel shame about those parts of you, then it follows that directing your attention there could bring up a memory in a way that feels entirely unwanted. We can see why paying any type of sustained attention to your genitals might be a very difficult thing to do. The fear of the pain accompanying that memory could even be the trigger for a dissociative response without your realizing it. You could also *choose* to actively engage that dissociation yourself in order to feel better.

The hormonal shifts that happen within our bodies occur without a conscious invitation to do so. It is likely that you did not ask for your menstrual cycle to occur exactly how it does or wish for perimenopause to start and continue the way it is. It may be upsetting to be confronted with these changes in the body, as they mirror a feeling of non-consent. This parallel feeling of non-consent may come up throughout menstruation, menopause, and fertility journeys.

Talia

Talia hears her girlfriend calling her name. It takes a fraction of a second, and Talia finds herself coming back into her body. As she responds, she gets the sense that she's zoned out. She and her girlfriend are familiar with what can sometimes happen to Talia—especially in moments of close connection, she can find she is mentally away from herself. She understands that dissociation was an adaptation that developed as a way to cope with childhood sexual trauma, and she has been successfully working at reducing her trauma responses in her adult years, but sometimes it still pops up.

Talia and her girlfriend adeptly reconnect. Later that evening over dinner, Talia mentions a new personal goal—she'd like to better manage some of her pelvic and vulvar pain. Her plan is to start tracking the intensity of these sensations of discomfort and to reconnect with her pelvic floor physical therapist once she has a few cycles of information. Talia wants to check in with her girlfriend before starting this type of tracking. She has noticed that doing work with her pelvic floor therapist as well as tracking more specific pain sensations can sometimes feel a bit overwhelming.

Talia's girlfriend tells her she is happy to be a support for her while she works on her pain and verbalizes all the care she has for Talia. For both, slowing things down and providing extra emotional support feels right. Talia plans to use the tracking category comfort *to articulate days in which she feels at peace with the support she has in her relationship.*

trapped

breathless

drowning

hazy

foggy

flashbacks

fuzzy

anxious

existential

anger

spiritual

numb

blank

disorganized

void

empty

stuck

panic

paralyzed

distracted

lost

slowed

floating

nightmares

heavy

lonely

questioning

sweating

despair

depression

queasy itchy icy

crampy

tingly

buzzy

agitation

small

tight

intrusive

tense

powerless

shame

tearful

restricted

hollow

TAKING CARE OF YOUR BODY IF YOU HAVE LIVED THROUGH TRAUMA

Reconnecting with the body at a pace determined entirely by *you* can alleviate the impacts of trauma. One way to do this is with mindfulness, the act of being connected to your own bodily sensations and practicing non-judgmental awareness of your body. These skills can lead to increased access to care and support.

Mindfulness can help take the power away from intrusive thoughts and out-of-control feelings. Tracking with non-judgmental body observation *is* mindfulness. We see how life-changing this practice is for our clients every day. While working on this particular skill, give yourself credit for the process. Celebrate yourself and your efforts. This is hard but valuable. Research shows that this really does work.

Dissociation and its companions, depersonalization (feeling like a stranger to yourself or as if you are observing yourself from a distance) and derealization (feeling that the world around you is not real), can significantly impact how people relate to and access care. People with lived traumatic experiences may seek help at lower rates, leading to decreased support and increased health risks. Higher rates of dissociation can lead to an increased risk of developing PTSD.

TRACKING PREP

What's working

If you notice numbness, emptiness, or any of these feelings of dissociation
in your own life, a starting place might be to approach this exercise
from a place of kindness. Your body and mind are working to protect you.

YOU GET TO DECIDE WHETHER THESE
SENSATIONS SERVE YOU OR NOT

One way dissociation has helped protect me is:

I feel _____ when remembering this.

How I feel about using dissociation as a coping method in the future:

TRACKING WITH TRAUMA

If you've experienced trauma, the truth is, cycle tracking may initially be difficult. *Being present is complicated when being numb has been your protection.* Listening to the body and observing pleasure, pain, and everything in between is an act of being present in many parts of that body.

You can still track if you've experienced trauma. You can still track if you live in this world full of trauma—*especially* if you live in this world.

If tracking is feeling daunting or even painful, this is so, so, so common. We recommend starting small and simple.

If any bit of what you are tracking feels stressful, then forget it for a while. Check it out later. Highlight what's accessible and build it into a new habit so tracking has the possibility to be joyful and rewarding. Many people find that it's most comfortable to start by tracking bleeding and only one other sensation. You would be amazed at how much of a resource just those two bits of information can be.

Especially when taking care of a body that has been through trauma, it is better to start tracking at a slow and comfortable pace.

TRACKING RECOMMENDATIONS:

1. Track less, track simple. Start by tracking no more than three categories. Try this for three cycles and then reevaluate whether the amount, level, and intensity of tracking feels good to you.

2. Start by experimenting with your use of the *comfort* category included in every chart from Day 1. As you get familiar with checking on your *comfort* on a daily basis, adding one additional *safety* category on top of *comfort* is optimal when creating a supportive foundation for trauma tracking.

3. Plan accordingly. Think about your day and plan for an extra cushion of time around tracking to take care of yourself before going back into your schedule.

4. Don't push too hard. You know what it feels like to experience overload related to trauma. There is no reason to flood yourself with these types of trauma responses. If you notice that you are dissociating, if you are feeling an intense emotion like anxiety or depression, or if you are finding tracking tiring or are avoiding it entirely, please listen to your system and take a break.

5. If you notice that tracking feels particularly hard or activating, you might want to check in with your body and ask yourself if you want to physically move it in any way. Move your body into a position that feels better. This can be a good reminder of agency.

    Remember, just the act of listening to your body is powerful.

TRACKING PREP

Identify your own tracking categories

We love collaborating with our clients to make tracking really *work* for them. One of our favorite parts of this process is narrowing down tracking categories from broad ideas to specific, descriptive, cogent sensations. Usually, when we ask people what they would like to track, they have general ideas such as pain, anxiety, and sex.

Pain can mean so many things. But when we focus in on descriptors with our clients, sensations like *stabbing*, *lightning*, *ripping*, *gnawing*, and *throbbing* mean so much more. *Anxiety* can turn into a *sour stomach* or *tight chest*. *Sex* can be so much more definite, like *turned on*, *excitement*, *more fantasies*, *feeling hot*, *release*.

Let's do the same here. Start with a general category and come up with some more illustrative, precise sensations below each. These sensations can be anything that have meaning to you. They do not have to be used by anyone else; they serve as *your* guide to what you want to learn about yourself. You can even use made-up words—these words need only evoke a recognizable, trackable feeling for you.

If you find yourself with writer's block, take a few minutes and use the body scan from page 29. Notice sensations within yourself and freely write some of what you are feeling.

Once you've found your sensations, these can be your tracking categories for your charts. Simply transfer your chosen sensations to your category lines and observe.

BROAD FEELING

Three of my own experiences I'd like to learn more about are:

-

-

-

SPECIFIC SENSATIONS

Using the *Broad Feeling* categories you've just identified, expand on how these experiences feel.

Some words that best describe how these feelings show up in my body, mind, emotions, or thoughts are:

-

-

-

CATEGORY

My first tracking category is:

1 Comfort

Looking at all of my Specific Sensations, *my favorite categories that I want to track are:*

2

3

4

Of these Specific Sensations, *certain ones seem to have more variability. The categories that I'd like to track the intensity of are:*

5

6

8.

Pain

When our pain is dismissed by those around us, we might learn to also dismiss it. When others take away the power of our language, when they don't hear our pain, we might learn to stop using that language even when speaking to ourselves. Without the words to describe and without the space to tell others how we feel, we can lose our voice.

In *The Pain Gap*, Anushay Hossain amplifies how coping with untreated pain can get even more complicated: "But what plagues me most is why I stayed so uncharacteristically quiet through it all. Why, when I insisted the painkillers weren't working and everyone was ignoring me, did I not once raise my voice? Why, after I was in surgery, was I so polite to the doctor who demanded I 'prove' my pain . . . ? Where was my voice[?]"

A knowledge gap (due to the historic lack of research on menstruating people) and a trust gap (due to providers not believing those people as much as they believe others) have created an insidious cycle of their own: our concerns about our bodies aren't taken seriously because providers generally lack in-depth knowledge about our bodies. This means that for many of us, the conditions we experience may be ignored, distrusted, or undervalued at higher rates because the medical profession doesn't know as much about them.

This also means that people reporting pain around their menstrual cycle are given psychosomatic explanations at higher rates than other patients. They are provided pain treatments and medications less frequently and at lower doses. They are often altogether dismissed before being given a diagnosis: "Sounds like period pain, take some ibuprofen." Within this cycle, funding for research around our biology continues to suffer. And so do we.

Normalizing and dismissing pain around the menstrual cycle, pregnancy, or menopause as "typical" experiences only serves to dismiss concerns and encourage people to tolerate pain they don't have to feel. We lose out on the opportunity for appropriate pain management.

The unknown schedule of this pain can create an independently occurring cycle—anxiety about feeling anxiety about pain. The connection between mood and physical sensations can complicate the experience of physical pain. When feelings like confusion, hopelessness, depression, or fear are present, as they often are, pain can take on a different quality. The intensity of these feelings can make the pain even more challenging.

This type of pain often makes sex feel different. Arousal and orgasm feel different. When sex feels different, so do we.

Pain with sex has even been shown to significantly impact a person's overall well-being, leading to a decreased quality of life, an increase in psychological pain and depression, and an interrupted sense of self.

There is a lack of comprehension in our society regarding the complexities of pelvic and genital pain. By understanding and tracking pain that is so wildly misunderstood and staggeringly misdiagnosed, you improve your chances of getting the care you deserve. By listening to your body and validating your own experiences, you gain the power to find the best treatment for you, to find collaborators, and to know that you are not alone and you don't have to be silent.

THROW AWAY THE SCALE

Finding ways to describe and identify different types of pain—surface and organ, specific and vague, chronic and acute—is a herculean effort. By finding a way to describe and convey pain, we have a better opportunity for successful collaboration and treatment with medical and care providers.

The complex experience of pain is personal, and the scales we use in an attempt to describe it often fall short. Not only is pain subjective, based on lived experiences and individual reference points, but our nervous systems are discrete and complex in ways that are difficult to comprehend.

Here's why labeling your pain on a scale of 1 to 10 can feel inadequate. Although attempts to create accessible measurements of pain continue, a time-bound, linear scale might not wholly capture the experience of chronic pain. It's subjective, with no agreed-upon baseline as a reference point for the person interpreting that 1-to-10 rating. Rating and interpretation both can be affected by several factors, including your personal pain threshold, how you were socialized to discuss your discomfort, and how pain was culturally treated when you were learning how to live in the world.

Self-reporting your pain in a vulnerable situation might instigate a trauma response—you might freeze, appease, or dissociate, finding it very hard to communicate how you feel without considering how the person hearing it might receive it. It might feel like losing your voice.

If we can't describe our pain fully to ourselves, it is impossible to imagine describing it to others who might be able to help, but that's where tracking can come in. Contextualizing sensations of pain and discomfort within cycle tracking can frame, identify, and even course-correct toward a treatment.

Consider the whole-body impact of discomfort when tracking pain. For example, dealing with genital pain may cause a lack of appetite even though that pain is not localized in the gastrointestinal tract. In this case, it would be helpful to also track reduced appetite when tracking your genital pain.

We love the alternative pain questionnaire created by Dr. Deborah Coady and Nancy Fish. It is a descriptive and comprehensive guide. We've included an adapted portion here. Their book, *Healing Painful Sex*, is a fantastic resource and was a vital part of research for this chapter.

WHAT IS THE QUALITY OF YOUR PAIN?

○ Burning
○ Itching/irritation
○ Throbbing
○ Aching

○ Stabbing
○ Sharp/shooting
○ Cramping

WHAT IS THE NATURE OF YOUR PAIN?

○ Generalized (you feel it all over)
○ Localized (it's coming from a very specific area)
○ Radiating (it starts in one area and spreads out from there)
○ Referred (it originates from one place but your body feels it somewhere else)
○ Constant (you feel it all the time)
○ Intermittent (you feel it sometimes)
○ Provoked (something touches you or something happens that causes the pain)
○ Unprovoked (the pain is there with no apparent trigger)

IF YOU CHECKED "PROVOKED," WHAT KINDS OF STIMULI MIGHT PROVOKE YOUR PAIN?

○ Sex (any type of sexual contact, including, but not limited to penetration)
○ Physical contact
○ Wearing underwear
○ Exercise

○ Anxiety
○ Lack of sleep
○ Sitting
○ Walking
○ Standing
○ Stretching

WHERE IS YOUR PAIN LOCATED? (SEE PAGES 237-245 FOR FULL ANATOMICAL DESCRIPTIONS)

○ Clitoris
○ Vestibule
○ Vagina
○ Cervix
○ Labia

○ Overall vulva
○ Anus
○ Upper thighs
○ Lower back
○ Abdomen

In our practices, we see the psychological impact of pain. We see people dealing with its invisible emotional weight. Our clients feel alone, ashamed, worried, and scared. Without space to talk about genital and sexual pain, they feel they have to stay silent and solve their own suffering. We see how this permeates all aspects of life, including sex and relationships. This is not a burden anyone should have to carry alone.

Ines

Ines knows how hard it was to get to where she is today—working with a team of specialists who take her pain seriously and have come up with a collaborative treatment plan for her endometriosis. She is beyond proud of herself for continuing to show up and advocate for care, even when it felt hopeless. Ines has learned so much about who she is as a person and how strong she can be, and she has identified her capacity to stand up for what she feels is right. Her values have become much more apparent to her. Ines still has a regular and active tracking practice as she makes ongoing choices about her endometriosis care, and she includes a category every cycle that reminds her of her agency, often using the tracking category comfort *to capture this sensation.*

TRACKING RECOMMENDATIONS:

1. Choose language extremely specific to your own pain for your tracking category.

2. The combination of intensity and your individual category provides a more robust picture of your body's experience through your cycle. Use the intensity bubbles to help strengthen your understanding of just how these sensations feel for you.

3. Add pleasure-tracking categories in order to have full context to your pain.

4. Challenge yourself to create two tracking categories that are impacted by your pain but are not direct pain sensations, like sleep, anxiety, or appetite.

SAVE YOURSELF A BIT OF TIME

These are some commonly misdiagnosed and underdiagnosed pain conditions. We've seen these come through our doors too many times, with our clients going years without clarity, despite all of their best efforts. We are sharing these with you because we have seen that identification gets you one crucial step closer to understanding your pain.

A diagnosis can be a name for your pain, but it doesn't always provide the full explanation as to why you are feeling the way you are. Some diagnoses can clarify *where* pain exists in your body, and some can clarify *what* may be causing it. Sometimes these conditions overlap, and we see clients with more than one at the same time—especially pelvic floor conditions, a common result of coping with these types of pain. We can't not tell you about them.

Location of Pain

These *location* diagnoses help you understand where your pain is felt. The causes of localized pain are diverse, and it is beneficial to explore potential reasons for the pain from a holistic perspective. These diagnoses are not necessarily an explanation of why the pain is happening but more a reference of where it's happening.

DYSPAREUNIA

— What is it?
Dyspareunia is a broad term for the experience of pain during genital sexual contact. It is not gender-specific and includes pain felt externally and internally. This is a medicalized term for painful sex that requires further diagnostic exploration. With continued inquiry this diagnosis may be specified into conditions like clitorodynia, vestibulodynia, or vulvodynia.

— How does it feel?
This term encompasses all experiences of physical discomfort and pain before, during, and after sexual contact in the genital region.

— How does it happen?

The causes of sexual pain are vast and holistic and can include many different combinations of experiences and feelings.

— What our clients say:

> "It feels like I physically cannot do what I want to do. I try really hard to push through the pain—it seems like a weakness. I want to be a good partner, but it is so hard to want to sexually connect because it hurts so badly. I don't feel in control of what's happening in my body."

CLITORODYNIA

— What is it?

Clitorodynia is a term for pain that occurs with the clitoris. Clitorodynia can be debilitating due to the complex of nerves located in this organ.

— How does it feel?

Clitoral pain can be experienced as an extreme sensitivity to touch or even clothing. The pain may also exist without any type of outside stimulation, meaning nothing has to touch you to feel the pain. You may experience this pain as short and sharp as well as lasting well beyond a moment of touch. It may feel burning or gnawing, hot-stabbing or sickening. Clitoral pain can also occur with orgasm.

— How does it happen?

The clitoris is an organ composed of muscle, blood vessels, and nerves. The external portion of the clitoris can be aggravated from outside sources and/or the internal organ can have nerve damage. Nerve damage can occur at the site of the clitoris or on the clitoral nervous pathway that leads to the spine.

Nerve damage or disruption in the broader pelvic region

Conditions that affect your nervous system, including herpes simplex virus

Vulvar dermatologic conditions

Circulatory and vascular differences

— What our clients say:

> " I'm afraid to feel pleasure because I'm not sure if that will be a time that I also feel pain. I'd rather stay away from it altogether. I can't figure out when it's going to happen, it feels so unpredictable."

INTERSTITIAL CYSTITIS

— What is it?

Interstitial cystitis is persistent and chronic bladder pain.

— How does it feel?

Many people experience pain in the bladder or a feeling of pressure in the lower abdomen. You may feel burning, tearing, cutting, or fiery sensations when urinating. More frequent or urgent trips to urinate may also be a symptom. For this reason, misdiagnosis of recurrent urinary tract infections (often with normal urine test results and no response to antibiotics) is quite common.

— How does it happen?

A few factors or a combination of factors may cause interstitial cystitis.

Previous medical or physical trauma

A possible inherited trait

An irritant that has gotten inside the bladder

Autoimmune conditions

— **What our clients say:**

> " I am so attuned to stuff being wrong 'down there' at this point
> of managing this chronic discomfort that I'm in a state of
> perpetual waiting to respond to pain. At any moment, I am ready
> to jump into action to try to prevent major overload and
> interruption of my life. I'm hyperaware of every sensation."

PELVIC FLOOR PAIN

— **What is it?**

The set of muscles that make up the pelvic floor are connected to many other body systems and provide direct support to the pelvis, including the bladder, bowels, rectum, anus, urethra, vagina, uterus, and spinal column. The pelvic floor muscles can exist in states of contraction or relaxation, and sometimes the muscles can even spasm uncontrollably. The tightness of the contraction or the looseness of the relaxation can create issues with the functioning of the systems the pelvic floor supports. Within the muscles and tissues of your pelvic floor, there is also an intricate network of nerves. These nerves send signals of sensation to our brains, allowing us to process touch, pleasure, and pain of the pelvic floor. The nerves in and around your internal organs process things like pain differently than the nerves of your skin and muscle. These nerves inside the body sense pain more broadly so it feels much less localized, which can present a challenge in diagnosis and understanding.

— **How does it feel?**

Because the pelvic floor muscles are connected to so many other body systems, changes in pelvic floor functioning can be expressed in reduced bladder or bowel control, back pain, a feeling of heaviness in the pelvis or genitals, or pain with genital penetration, among many other sensations. When nerves are compressed or damaged, pain signals may be sent to the brain that are much more difficult to decipher. For instance, your brain may be getting a signal from a nerve that there is tissue damage and injury that needs attention, but, in reality, that nerve

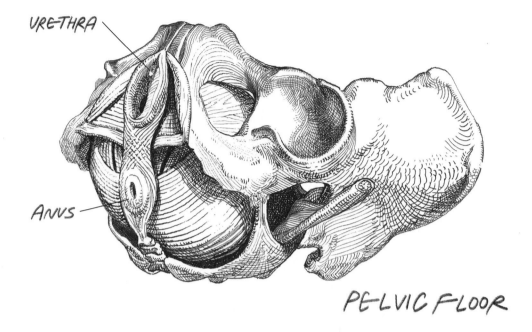

URETHRA

ANUS

PELVIC FLOOR

is pinched or compressed, while there is no tissue damage. Your brain may have a hard time identifying that sensation as nerve pain. Pain may also be felt in surrounding physical areas if they overcompensate for pelvic floor dysregulation.

— How does it happen?
Pelvic floor pain can occur as a result of many different experiences. Some are:

Previous medical, physical, emotional, or sexual pain and/or trauma

Other coexisting pelvic pain disorders (including everything you see in this chapter)

Years lived

Physical injury, heavy lifting, or trauma

Chronic constipation or diarrhea

Giving birth (vaginally or via surgery)

— **What our clients say:**

> " It feels like my insides are falling out of my bottom.
> I can't sneeze without peeing my pants. I didn't know
> my pelvic floor had so much to do with my bowels.
> Everything feels so heavy. "

VESTIBULODYNIA

— **What is it?**

Vestibulodynia refers to pain at the genital opening. The vestibule is the tissue in between the labia and the vagina. This type of pain is often called vaginismus. We believe *vestibulodynia* works better in this case to clarify and identify the cause of your pain.

Irritation, inflammation, and thinning of the vestibule can occur with or without physical touch or provocation.

Pain with penetration or attempted penetration can cause involuntary muscle spasms to occur at the opening of the vagina. These muscle spasms can occur in response to any type of pain from penetration—including a pelvic exam, the attempted insertion of a menstruation product, or a desired sexual touch from another person, a toy, or yourself. This can happen at any point in a person's life and can come and go.

— **How does it feel?**

This is a painful experience that can be felt on a scale of intensity. It may feel like tolerable discomfort with penetration, or it may prevent penetration entirely. It may be consistent with all attempts at penetration, or it may feel better or worse on different occasions. You may feel like there is a "block" or a wall inside the genitals, stopping something from entering, or you may feel like the internal genitals are too tight, too small, or too narrow. You may have a feeling that there is something inside you that is in the way or that your body will not let you do what you want. Emotional frustration, anxiety, and low mood can be logical reactions to the experience of your body doing something that you don't want it to do.

— **How does it happen?**

The causes of vestibulodynia are individualized and often challenging to definitively identify. Even though it may be hard to immediately pinpoint cause, this diagnosis can still be a useful step in helping with your pain. Here are some possible experiences that might lead to vestibular pain:

Previous medical, physical, emotional, or sexual pain and/or trauma

Other coexisting pelvic pain disorders (including everything you see in this chapter)

Nerve damage or disruption in the pelvic region

Pelvic floor conditions

Conditions that affect your nervous system, including herpes simplex virus

Possible inherited trait

— **What our clients say:**

> " It feels like there is a wall and there is nothing getting past it.
> It's like my insides have closed a door and I can't get it open.
> I can't really use tampons anymore. When I have sex it feels like
> nothing will move beyond a certain physical point inside me.
> I feel so guilty that these situations turn into an
> ordeal that has to be discussed."

VULVODYNIA

— **What is it?**

Vulvodynia is pain experienced at and around the vulva, including the clitoris and the vaginal opening. Vulvodynia is also sometimes categorized as one of the complex regional pain syndromes (CRPS) that impact other parts of the body.

— How does it feel?

You may feel your vulva throb, ache, or feel stinging, itchy, burning, raw, or swollen. You may notice discomfort when the vulva is touched in any way, including by clothing or underwear. The sensation may be persistent, only in response to touch or physical irritation, or it may even come and go randomly without a stimulus correlation.

— How does it happen?

As with all *location* diagnoses, the causes of vulvodynia are often challenging to distinguish. It might require some extra investigation on your part, but there are many avenues to explore.

Possible experiences that may lead to this condition are:

Previous medical, physical, emotional, or sexual pain and/or trauma

Other coexisting pelvic pain disorders (including everything you see in this chapter)

Nerve damage or disruption in the pelvic region

Conditions that affect your nervous system, including herpes simplex virus

Personal environmental factors

Allergic reactions

Vaginal infections—you may want to explore bacterial vaginosis (BV) or yeast/candida

— What our clients say:

" Getting any type of pelvic exam with a speculum is so painful. I notice that I postpone getting my annual for as long as I can. Paps are the worst; it feels like fire touching my skin. I spend a lot of time trying to figure out what exactly might trigger it, and when. "

Shape of Pain

These *shape* diagnoses refer to a specific cause of your pain. A structural condition has been identified that is directly linked to the pain you feel.

GENITAL TISSUE DRYING, THINNING, AND INFLAMMATION

— What is it?

Also known as atrophic vaginitis or vaginal atrophy, genital tissue drying, thinning, and inflammation refers to the impact of reduced estrogen on internal vaginal tissue and the urinary tract. Reduced estrogen can thin the internal vaginal walls and reduce production of lubricating body fluids, making the tissue less flexible and more susceptible to tearing and bleeding.

— How does it feel?

People experiencing genital tissue drying, thinning, and inflammation might notice sensitivity, discomfort, tenderness, and pain with vaginal penetration as well as a feeling of vaginal dryness or burning. You might describe the feeling as scratchy or stinging, burning, stabbing, splitting, or ripping. You might feel a change in the texture and moisture of the genital tissue to the touch. If there are urinary tract symptoms, you might notice an increase in frequency, urgency, and discomfort with urination as well as urinary tract infections. You might notice genital fluids that don't feel like your normal. You may notice bleeding or spotting after penetration of any type. Discomfort might be felt when inserting a tampon or cup during the bleeding phase of menstruation. It also might be felt when simply sitting or walking. You might feel it when a pelvic floor physical therapist, obstetrician, gynecologist, or midwife touches you or begins to insert a gelled, gloved finger.

— How does it happen?

Shifts in estrogen levels are highly individual. However, there are many common causes of reduced estrogen levels that have been connected to these tissue symptoms.

Perimenopause and postmenopause hormone changes (doctors may refer to this change in tissue in the context of menopause as genitourinary syndrome of menopause, or GSM)

Some hormonal contraceptives can lead to a decrease in estrogen

Radiation, chemotherapy, and hormonal treatments for cancer or other conditions

Lactation, bodyfeeding or nursing a baby

— What our clients say:

> " I felt like my vagina dried up after I had my baby.
> Even something as gentle as wiping with toilet paper
> made my skin feel like it was ripping."

ENDOMETRIOSIS

— What is it?

Endometriosis is a chronic condition in which the endometrial cells that typically exist inside the uterus also exist in other places in the body. During menstruation, when endometrial cells typically leave the uterus during the bleeding phase, the endometrial cells that exist elsewhere in the body cause inflammation cyclically and can potentially cause fibrous scar tissue adhesions wherever they exist. This can lead to chronic pain or muscular or organ dysfunction wherever the cells may be located in the body. A very similar condition, adenomyosis, occurs when endometrial cells grow into the uterine muscle.

— How does it feel?

You may experience sharp or dull or rhythmic or consistent pains in your body during your bleeding phase. Some people experience no pain. Most commonly, endometriosis is found and experienced in the abdomen around the uterus, or on the bladder, colon, and intestines. Endometriosis can be felt with gastrointestinal symptoms like bloating, cramping, diarrhea, constipation, feelings of swelling or pressure, stiffness around the bladder and abdomen, and internal muscular pain and pulling. Sometimes the pain levels are so high that people may faint or vomit from the discomfort.

— How does it happen?

The causes of endometriosis are still being explored. What we now know is that endometriosis may be a result of a few different experiences:

A possible inherited trait

Physical trauma caused by abdominal surgeries

— What our clients say:

> " I'm just so exhausted by this seemingly inevitable pain. So much of my life revolves around whether it is active. It's so hard to function sometimes."

FIBROIDS

— What are they?

Uterine fibroids are collections of fibrous, noncancerous tissue in or on the uterus. They are pretty common and can vary in size from less than 1 millimeter to large enough to fill the abdomen.

— How does it feel?

People with fibroids may experience heavy bleeding or clotting with menstruation, as the uterus has a trickier time trying to coordinate its muscles to empty itself. You may also experience pain, discomfort, pressure, aching, and cramping from the size of a fibroid pushing on internal organs, muscles, and ligaments. While many fibroids go unnoticed and do not cause any pain, some may warrant surgical removal or medical treatment.

— How does it happen?

The causes of fibroids are unknown. We do know that estrogen and progesterone are present in the cells that make up fibroids.

Risk factors and correlation links are still being researched, but current data puts certain populations at higher risk, including people of color.

As many as 80 percent of uteruses develop fibroids by the time someone is fifty years old. Because estrogen and progesterone are present in the cells of fibroids, they may shrink later in life with the hormonal changes that occur at menopause.

— What our clients say:

*" My belly was so 'pooched out,' I wondered if I was pregnant.
Deep penetration is truly uncomfortable,
and I avoid it as much as I can."*

VULVAR DERMATOLOGIC CONDITIONS

— What is it?

The skin on your vulva can develop dermatological conditions in the same way as the skin on the rest of your body. Some conditions that cause discomfort include eczema, psoriasis, folliculitis, contact dermatitis, greater vestibular gland cysts, lichen simplex chronicus, lichen sclerosus, and lichen planus.

— How does it feel?

You may experience burning or itching sensations. Your skin may feel itchy, bumpy, scaly, wrinkled, hot, raw, or swollen. These sensations can be localized or encompass the whole vulva.

— How does it happen?

The causes of vulvar dermatologic conditions are unique to all of us and a combination of factors may contribute.

May be inherited

Tissue damage or irritation

Contact with chemicals, fragrances, fabrics, soaps, lotions, lubricants, and other substances that cause irritation

Allergic reaction

— **What our clients say:**

> " I couldn't even wear underwear without discomfort, itching, and stinging. Sex felt off the table. I could hardly stand to sit still when it was really bad."

TRACKING PREP

Identifying sensations

What does it feel like to be fluent in your body's language?

We find that a valuable first step toward identifying your body's
sensations is defining your own vocabulary. Your body gives
you cues that let you know how and what you feel.

IMAGINE YOUR MIND IS A ROOM

There is a door you walked through to get there. In the room there are two chairs.

If I were to draw it, my mind's room looks like:

YOU ARE IN THE ROOM

You sit in one chair and realize that facing you in the other chair is . . . you. Really visualize yourself, look directly into your own eyes.

As I sit in my chair and see myself sitting across from me . . .

I notice that my facial expression is:

My posture looks:

My age is:

Ask the person sitting across from you, "If I could do anything for you right now, what would it be? If I could better understand anything about how you feel right now, what would it be?"

The response I get is:

Your time in the room is coming to an end. Look at yourself in the chair across from you and thank yourself for your time. Thank yourself for sharing. Say farewell and walk out the door on the other side of the room. Close the door.

Some of the more surprising or standout feelings I learned from myself in the room are:

These feelings are a fantastic foundation for building body awareness and sensation tracking ideas.

A feeling I would like to expand is:

A feeling I would like to change is:

A new feeling I would like to have is:

9.

Cycle Phases

When we are taught about menstruation, it's within a heteronormative context of having a baby. It's called the *reproductive* system, and the exploration of human biology often doesn't go much further than that. When we are taught about pregnancy, we learn about ovulation. Outside school, mainstream dialogue about the cycle is all about "biohacking" or "balancing" or "modifying" your hormones.

To support and encourage the awareness of our bodies *all* the time, not just when, or if, we are thinking about fertility, we like to use a definition of menstruation that doesn't focus on reproduction at all. To aid a deeper understanding of our bodies, we get curious about what the body is communicating instead of trying to "hack" it. The menstrual cycle is a series of biological events that occur in response to hormonal changes in the body. It's a common and critical bodily function, with nearly 1.8 billion people around the world menstruating at any given time.

Let's look at it through a different lens.

In the simplest of terms, there are four primary events that occur in the menstrual cycle as a result of an exciting hormonal orchestra. These four primary events are bleeding (the menstrual phase), preparing to ovulate (the follicular phase), ovulating (the ovulatory phase), and preparing to bleed again (the luteal phase).

Menstrual *is based on the Latin word for* month, *even though we know people's cycles vary widely outside of a monthly calendar.*

Follicular *is based on the Latin word for* little sac *to describe the sac (follicle) that holds an egg cell.*

Ovulatory *is based on the Latin word for* egg, *which is* ova.

Luteal *is based on the Latin word for* yellow, *which describes the appearance of the follicle after it releases an egg cell.*

Here's an overview of each phase:

Menstrual Phase. *Tracking your menstrual cycle typically begins with the bleeding phase, during which the uterine lining separates from the uterus and disintegrates. Then the body pushes the egg cell, blood, and disintegrated uterine tissues out of the uterus, through the cervix, and out through the vagina.*

Follicular Phase. *The body prepares follicles, or fluid-filled cases, inside the ovaries. The ovary matures a set of follicles each cycle, and they go on to act as protectors and transporters of egg cells. The number of follicles that mature is different for every person, but typically only one of the largest and strongest follicles will go on to the next phase, and the other follicles will disintegrate in place. During the follicular phase, the uterus plumps up its interior lining again, having just emptied itself out by bleeding in the menstrual phase.*

Ovulatory Phase. *The largest, strongest, most mature follicle from the ovary now releases an egg cell. The egg cell travels through the uterine tube and into the uterus.*

Luteal Phase. *The luteal phase takes place between ovulation and bleeding. The follicle that once held the egg cell changes in structure and function. It's now called a corpus luteum, and while its previous job was to protect the egg cell, its new job is to continue to plump the uterine lining through producing hormones. This prepares the body to bleed again. Once the corpus luteum has completed its job, it also disintegrates in place.*

If sperm is in the picture, these phases can look different:

Ovulatory Phase. *If sperm is present and combines with the egg cell, they then continue to travel together toward the uterus.*

Luteal Phase. *The egg and sperm continue their journey into the uterus.*

Implantation. *When the combined egg and sperm cells land in the uterus, they embed themselves in the plumped uterine lining. If pregnancy continues, the menstrual phases pause.*

After your body has completed the four phases, it starts the process all over, beginning again with the menstrual phase. Many menstruating people assume that they ovulate on Day 14 of a cycle, but this statistic is based on outdated, oversimplified averages. Even if you have a fairly regular cycle, ovulation and cycle phases can vary each time.

Ramona

Ramona discovered a pattern through her tracking and identified the ovulatory and luteal phases as key to her workflow and artistic expression. Without being too "life-hacky," she makes choices for herself based on how she has learned these cycle phases make her feel. These two cycle phases are the most relevant to her, and she doesn't think much about the other two. Ramona uses the comfort *tracking category to signify days in which she feels secure in her sense of her cyclical pattern. Even if she is having an "off" day, she can still access comfort as she knows this feeling won't last forever. She allows herself to take care of her needs at that time in her cycle, knowing that this will shift as she moves into the next phase.*

Each cycle can look different from person to person, and the timing of each phase can vary, as can the sensations you feel from phase to phase or cycle to cycle. Even if they feel inconsistent or random, the sensations in your body often work in patterns, and understanding the major phases of menstruation can help you prepare and support your body through these cycles.

10.

Hormones

LISTENING TO YOUR HORMONES

Your body is made up of intricate pathways, woven into systems, each designed to help a part of you function. Your body's cells produce hormones, which act as your body's traveling messengers, telling your systems what to do and encouraging these systems to work together.

You may have heard about ways to correct your hormones. We like to consider hormones a bit differently. If hormones really are messengers in our bodies, then we find that it feels helpful to listen to them instead of changing what they are trying to tell you. The way hormones show up in our lives can be treated as a symptom or as a bigger conversation.

What does your body need more of?

Hormones are essential to your physical functions like metabolism, energy levels, sleep, and arousal, as well as your emotions, thoughts, and feelings. Hormonal shifts have been linked to changes in mood and how intensely mental health conditions are felt. With our clients, we regularly see that the symptom severity of many psychological states like depression, anxiety, and OCD changes with those shifts.

Your hormonal system, also known as your endocrine system, has glands located throughout your entire body. Those glands make and release hormones that help you function all day, every day. There are also hormones outside your body that can be introduced into the body through hormone replacement therapies (HRTs), androgen suppressants, therapeutic testosterone, hormonal birth control, or other therapeutic contexts. Whether produced inside your body or outside your body, every hormone can impact the way you feel each and every day.

Your body responds to the world around you. This means that your body creates hormones tailored to your life. Because of this relationship, everyone's cycle is unique.

Nasreen

Nasreen has been using a urine ovulation test to help her identify her fertile window. The test she has been using shows a smiley face when it detects peak luteinizing hormone (LH). Each cycle, she waits for the smiley face, times penetrative sex accordingly, and doesn't get pregnant. During her evaluation with her midwife, she learns about other methods to observe ovulation, including different urine LH tests that use numbers to indicate hormonal levels instead of smiley faces, body fluid observation, basal body temperature (BBT), and cues related to how she feels.

After three cycles of tracking, Nasreen becomes aware of a few patterns. Her LH levels rise and fall multiple times a cycle. Nasreen also has multiple instances of slippery body fluids during just one cycle and she sees no sustained increase in her BBT. She's also surprised that the other sensations she has chosen to track don't seem to have a pattern with her LH, body fluids, or temperatures.

After sharing her charts with her midwife, Nasreen and her provider discover that she has not been ovulating. As she feels relief that she finally understands her cycle patterns, she is able to revisit the idea of peace and rest within herself. Nasreen takes this as a sign to take her mental health seriously as she continues to try to conceive.

Tests like an ovulation predictor kit with a smiley face are useful, but remember, hormones are an interwoven orchestra, so isolating one flute note on a Tuesday at six p.m. doesn't tell us what the song sounds like. This is helpful information and understanding hormonal values has great benefits, but it's not always enough.

WHO'S TALKING

At any given time, there are around fifty active hormones in your body. During the menstrual cycle, five key hormones help move the body through the cycle's core phases: follicle stimulating hormone (FSH), luteinizing hormone (LH), estrogens, progesterone, and testosterone. Serotonin, dopamine, and norepinephrine are also closely intertwined with the four main phases. These are by no means the *only* hormones present during the menstrual cycle; rather, they're the ones that tend to be most closely connected to your menstrual phases.

Estrogens

— **What are they?**
Estrogens are a bundle of hormones produced primarily by the ovaries and adrenal glands. There are four types of estrogen hormones: estradiol, estriol, estetrol, and estrone. Estradiol is the most common during a person's menstruating years, while estriol and estetrol are active during pregnancy and estrone is most present after menopause.

— **What do they do?**
Estrogens have two important jobs: to signal ovulation and to tell the uterus when it's time to thicken and release its lining. Increased estrogens can also boost other hormones like serotonin, dopamine, and norepinephrine, which are all responsible for mood and arousal.

— **What effect can they have?**
Changing levels of estrogens can impact many things, including body shape,

body size, temperature, sweating, mood, skin, hair, digestion, and chest tenderness, and they can also impact other body parts, including blood vessels, bones, and the brain. Because estrogens impact cortisol regulation, these hormonal shifts can also affect stress levels.

— When do they show up in my cycle?

They're lowest during the bleeding phase of the menstrual cycle, they peak during ovulation, and they lower during the luteal phase. The start of the follicular phase is often marked by a dip in estradiol. As follicles develop, they produce more estradiol, which helps rebuild and thicken the uterine lining—replacing the lining that you just released during your last bleeding phase.

— How can I track them?

Estrogens impact a range of bodily sensations and functions. Body fluids and genital lubrication, for example, fluctuate depending on levels of estrogens. While the social stigma around genital lubrication or dryness causes many to avoid observing body fluids, recognizing fluid shifts can help you identify ever-changing estrogen levels and better manage the corresponding bodily sensations throughout your cycle. On the whole, estrogen levels fluctuate during perimenopause and menopause. Estrogens decrease in postmenopause. Estrogens can also be monitored and measured through blood, urine, and saliva.

Follicle stimulating hormone (FSH)

— What is it?

FSH is a hormone produced by the pituitary gland that travels through the bloodstream to the ovaries.

— What does it do?

FSH triggers follicles to start growing.

— What effect can it have?

It can affect your mood, energy, and even appetite. Because FSH is responsible for producing and regulating follicles in the ovaries, the amount of the hormone can cause a differing number of follicles to develop.

— When does it show up in my cycle?
FSH is most present during the follicular phase. It peaks prior to ovulation and is at its lowest during the luteal phase.

— How can I track it?
While it's not easy to monitor FSH directly through cycle tracking, monitoring other sensations you feel around ovulation can give you insight into this hormone's cycle. FSH can also be monitored and measured through blood and urine.

Luteinizing hormone (LH)

— What is it?
LH is another hormone produced by the pituitary gland.

— What does it do?
LH is the hormone that signals the chosen follicle to release its egg cell in a cycle. It's generally steady throughout your cycle and peaks right before ovulation.

— What effect can it have?
In conjunction with other hormones, the peak and fall of LH within a cycle may affect mood, arousal, and energy. Irregular levels of LH may impact the ability to ovulate.

— When does it show up in my cycle?
The body experiences a surge of LH during ovulation, which helps the egg cell reach its peak maturity.

— How can I track it?
You can monitor LH through blood or urine with an ovulation predictor kit (OPK), which consists of paper test strips that you put into a cup you've urinated in. The

strip changes color depending on the amount of LH present in the body. You can also track ovulation retrospectively by analyzing your basal body temperatures (BBT) from a past cycle. (For more information on BBT, see chapter 16.) Additionally, tracking personalized sensations around ovulation can clue you in to when LH might be at its peak.

Progesterone

— What is it?
Progesterone is produced by the corpus luteum, the transformed follicle that just released an egg cell from the ovary.

— What does it do?
Progesterone plays a key role in the menstrual cycle by managing the lining that builds inside the uterus. It has also been shown to impact mood, build new bone, interplay with brain function and memory, and affect gastrointestinal function, including constipation, irritable bowel syndrome, and metabolism.

— What effect can it have?
Progesterone may cause chest tenderness and impact mood shifts, including anxiety and depression. Reduced levels of progesterone have been linked to early pregnancy loss, difficulty conceiving, and irregular menstrual cycles.

— When does it show up in my cycle?
Progesterone increases between the ovulation and bleeding phases.

— How can I track it?
The presence of progesterone can raise your basal body temperature, so you can track progesterone retrospectively by analyzing previous temperatures. (For more information on BBT, see chapter 16.) Levels in the body fluctuate as perimenopause begins and decrease in postmenopause. Progesterone can also be monitored and measured through blood, urine, and saliva.

Testosterone

— **What is it?**

Testosterone is a hormone produced by the ovaries and the adrenal glands.

— **What does it do?**

Testosterone significantly affects mood and sex drive, as well as energy and bone and muscle mass.

— **What effect can it have?**

Testosterone helps grow, maintain, and repair genital organs. It can affect hair growth and skin changes.

— **When does it show up in my cycle?**

Testosterone peaks during the ovulation phase.

— **How can I track it?**

Tracking your mood and feelings of sexual arousal, connection, and desire may help you identify the presence of this hormone during your cycle. Testosterone levels in the body fluctuate as perimenopause begins and decrease in post-menopause. Testosterone can be monitored and measured through blood, urine, and saliva.

Serotonin, dopamine, and norepinephrine

— **What are they?**

These hormones are believed to be central regulators of your mood. When estrogen levels increase, so do levels of serotonin, dopamine, and norepinephrine, which is a reason why some experience mood shifts as they move through their menstrual cycle.

— **What do they do?**

Serotonin is connected to sleep patterns, arousal, anxiety, and pain, while dopamine influences happiness, focus, concentration, and motivation. Norepinephrine influences your heart rate and can impact alertness, arousal, and decision-making ability.

— What effect can they have?
Because these hormones are so closely linked to mood, changing levels have been correlated with anxiety, depression, or trouble concentrating or making decisions.

— When do they show up in my cycle?
Because of the regular interplay between estrogens and serotonin, dopamine, and norepinephrine, as well as environmental influences that impact mood, these hormones are present throughout the cycle to varying degrees.

— How can I track them?
Identifying the sensations you feel around your mood may be a helpful starting point for creating a cycle-tracking system related to these neurotransmitters.

THE SYSTEMS YOUR HORMONES ARE TALKING ABOUT

All body systems are interconnected, and the genital system can illuminate the status and well-being of seemingly unrelated body parts and systems. Estrogen and progesterone receptors are found throughout the body and in most major body systems. Because these receptors are so omnipresent, you may find that you feel your body responds to hormonal shifts in systems that you might not expect.

Cardiovascular System

The cardiovascular system includes your heart and blood vessels, which all help regulate your body temperature and send oxygen and nutrients throughout your body.

You might find your heart beating slightly faster during the ovulatory and luteal phases and slightly slower during the bleeding and follicular phases. You may notice temperature changes during different hormonal phases or when your body is going through broader hormonal changes.

Digestive System

The digestive system, which includes your mouth, esophagus, stomach, and intestines, helps your body absorb nutrients and eliminate waste.

Right before the bleeding phase begins, hormones in your body send out a message to relax. This supports the uterus in pushing out its lining. This may also impact the tissues in your intestines, which may change how your poop feels and affect your poop schedule.

Hormonal shifts naturally occurring throughout life changes can affect how your gastrointestinal system feels and functions. Many genital and pelvic pain conditions, like endometriosis and pelvic floor pain, can also impact your digestive system and have been linked to gastrointestinal cramping, changes in bowel movements, appetite, and generalized sensations such as nausea.

Endocrine System

The endocrine system is made up of your hormones and the glands that produce them. These hormones regulate all sorts of body functions, including growth, development, and managing your metabolism. It's a huge network of communication within the body, which can impact your mood, physical comfort, resiliency, arousal, and more sensations than we could ever list. This won't be news to you; these hormone receptors are found all over your body and these messengers can change the way you feel.

Integumentary System

The integumentary system forms the outermost layer of the body, including the skin, hair, nails, and the glands that make oil and sweat.

Cyclical hormonal changes have been linked to significant changes in skin thickness, elasticity, water-carrying capacity, wound healing, and protective capability of the skin, as well as changes in texture and volume of hair. When observing skin, don't forget to include the skin around your genitals. This includes your vulva.

There are many times that hormonal shifts may result in what feels like a pretty dramatic change in the integumentary system. Let's look at hair—head hair, nipple hair, facial hair, all sorts of body hair. You may experience hair growth during pregnancy, hair loss and thinning connected to postpartum or perimenopause, and full-body hair changes connected to PCOS.

Lymphatic System

The lymphatic system, an integral part of the greater immune system, is a complex network that protects the body from infections and outside elements that may harm the body.

Hormonal shifts during the menstrual cycle can lead to people reporting a pattern of sickness or that their chronic conditions are cyclically exacerbated.

We often see clients identifying the presence of an autoimmune condition—when the body's lymphatic system attacks healthy cells—during times of big hormonal change, such as with the onset of menstruation or pregnancy.

Muscular System

The muscular system is made up of more than six hundred skeletal muscles that provide mobility to your body by attaching to your bones, as well as hundreds more smooth muscle tissues that provide mobility to your organs.

Hormonal shifts during the menstrual cycle can impact the strength and endurance of certain muscles within the body, which may impact your comfort with exercise or body movement at certain times of your cycle.

Nervous System

The nervous system is made up of the brain, nerves, and spinal cord and oversees sensory input and output to the rest of your body. The pelvic region holds an intricate system of nerves, and as a result, pelvic sensations can be intense when these nerves are damaged or compressed.

Nerve sensation can physically feel electric, zingy, and painful. It can be persistent or isolated to shorter moments. Emotionally, the stress, trauma, and discomfort we feel is also held within the nervous system. Some studies have shown that the social stress that often accompanies menstruation—in the form of interpersonal interactions, resiliency levels, or fatigue-related stress—has a direct impact on the nervous system, even to the point of being a risk factor for hormonal mood conditions.

Respiratory System

The respiratory system is responsible for delivering oxygen to the body and removing carbon dioxide from the body.

The menstrual cycle has been shown to have an impact on breathing quality. This may show up as an increase in coughing or chest discomfort, or, if you are managing a chronic condition such as asthma, you may notice higher-intensity symptoms and needs.

Skeletal System

When people are born, the skeletal system is made up of 270 bones. Some of those bones fuse over time, resulting in a total of 206 bones. These bones offer support and protect your organs.

Bones are storage sites for minerals (like calcium) and fats. Hormonal shifts have been linked to significant changes in bone health, most prominently osteoporosis. Osteoporosis has been referenced as inevitable with age, a mindset arguably rooted in the systemic dismissal of hormonally related health conditions. We now know that bone density is directly connected to estrogen levels, and estrogen helps in calcium absorption. A drop in estrogen during perimenopause is correlated with a decrease in bone density.

This is another example of a condition that is highlighted in moments of hormonal change, has multiple treatment options, and may require self-knowledge and self-advocacy to support.

Urinary System

The urinary system includes the bladder, ureters, kidneys, and urethra. This system filters blood to produce and release urine and other waste.

Hormonal shifts have been linked to changes in urinary system health, which can then impact the vaginal microbiome, pH levels, and pelvic floor functioning. Sometimes these changes can lead to painful or difficult sensations in the urethra, vagina, or pelvic floor region, or when urinating.

HANDING YOUR HORMONES A MEGAPHONE

Links between the hormonal cycle and many physical conditions are known, but more research needs to be done. The health field knows that these things are correlated, but we don't yet know the full reasons.

Cycle tracking is a critical tool. It's like giving your hormones a megaphone.

When hormone levels shift, whether it is during the menstrual cycle, pregnancy, postpartum, or perimenopause, the way certain emotional and physical conditions feel can change. For example, symptoms of asthma have been shown to differ at changing points in the menstrual cycle.

Some conditions that have been linked to varying levels of hormones include autoimmune conditions like Hashimoto's, multiple sclerosis, and lupus, as well as cancer, cardiovascular disease, infertility, ovarian hyperstimulation, diabetes, irritable bowel syndrome, and psychiatric conditions.

The fact that hormonal cycles can illuminate how these conditions show up in your body can be a major opportunity. The needs of our bodies change at different points in our lives. This is part of the human experience. Paying attention to our bodies provides us with opportunities to understand how to best support those changes.

11.

Charting Your Cycle

Our cycle-tracking goals with our clients over the years have been pretty straightforward—we want to better understand how their hormonal cycles impact their bodies and minds. We struggled to find a tracking tool that wasn't overcomplicated, oversimplified, or missing this jackpot intersection of mental health and the body. We love this system because it works.

We've refined three charting themes as the connection points to achieve these goals. We use these to structure our work with our clients and with ourselves, and now we're sharing them with you:

> *Your individual-to-you hormonal biomarkers*
>
> *Your sensation frequency and intensity*
>
> *Your broader life context*

Let's walk through the charts together and find out what's included in your chart and why, and of course, how to use it.

WHAT'S IN YOUR CHART

As the expert, you get to decide exactly what the charts on the following pages look like. We've established the scaffolding for each cycle, but you're in charge of deciding which categories to track, how to track them, and for how long you want to track.

The horizontal axis (top and bottom) of the chart is marked by the day of your cycle. The vertical axis (left side) of the chart is composed of everything you will be tracking. These are your hormonal biomarker anchors and your self-defined categories to track throughout your cycle.

YOUR INDIVIDUAL-TO-YOU HORMONAL BIOMARKERS

Basal Body Temperature and Body Fluids

To start you off, we've included basal body temperature and body fluids as categories in every single chart because they serve as core signals of hormonal changes. These biomarkers are here to anchor your cycle investigation. Charting these hormonal biomarkers can identify not only what hormones are more or less present at certain times in your cycle, but also how that shows up for you. No algorithms, predictions, or generalizations. This is your baseline, individualized to you.

Basal body temperature and changing body fluids can signify hormonal fluctuations so subtle that without attention they can go completely unnoticed. One of the most accessible and accurate ways to observe these hormonal changes is by taking a daily basal body temperature and noticing body fluid qualities.

While it is also possible to assess hormone levels through blood, saliva, and urine testing, this form of testing only tells us how much of a hormone is present at a particular time and point in your body. Evaluating *quantitative* values of hormones more frequently can give *qualitative* insight into how your body functions. In other words, isolated lab testing can tell us great information about a blip in time, but daily tracking of basal body temperature and body fluids also lets us delve into the "So what?" of it all, detailing how your body is responding to these hormone levels in action, day to day.

If you have regular and similar-length cycles and dependable body fluid changes, you may find that taking your basal body temperature for only three to six cycles provides ample data for reference. After tracking for a handful of cycles you may be able to recognize other biomarkers of hormonal shifts that occur in a pattern with those temperatures.

For instance, some people are better able to use body fluid fluctuations to gauge shifts in hormones after recognizing their consistent presence alongside these temperature shifts. If you notice variability in your cycle length or big shifts in the sensations you are tracking, returning to temperature monitoring might help you understand potential hormonal fluctuations that are at the root of these changes.

For more information on body fluids and basal body temperature, see chapters 15 and 16, "Body Fluids" and "Basal Body Temperature (BBT)."

Your Categories and Filling in the Bubbles

In each chart you will see six rows of bubbles: four rows have one bubble per day and the two rows below have three bubbles per day. Rows 1–4 allow you to track the absence or presence of your sensations. Rows 5–6 allow you to rate on a scale of 1 to 3 the intensity of a sensation. You've already finished your tracking prep exercise to identify your personal tracking categories on page 87. Now it's time to use them. Write the categories you would like to track this cycle on the *category* lines on your chart.

YOUR SENSATION FREQUENCY AND INTENSITY

Do you want to understand when, or if, your categories are showing up in your life? Do you want to understand how intense they feel? Use the bubbles accordingly.

Rows 1–4 offer you a bubble to fill in the presence and absence of something, so place those categories there. When looking to investigate the intensity of a sensation, place those categories in line 5 or 6.

When a category is present, fill in the bubble in rows 1–4.

When intensity fluctuates, fill in more or less of the bubbles in rows 5 and 6.

Every chart starts with the category called *comfort* on line 1. We've done this intentionally, as this is a wildly helpful category to track. The simple act of noticing when you feel grounded, safe, at ease—comfort—can be a powerful support to tracking anything you might be exploring. This category is not mandatory, of course, as your charts are yours to use however you'd like. We have included this because we have seen just how clarifying it can be for ourselves and all the people we have worked with.

YOUR BROADER LIFE CONTEXT

Some of your categories may not be sensations but instead tracking habits, activities, or routines. This is your broader life context. When you look at categories of things that occur *outside* your body, it can help define more about what's going on *inside*. You'll be able to notice whether certain categories are in line with hormone shifts or not.

CHARTING YOUR FIRST CYCLE

Okay. Let's do it.

STEP 1. Identify where to start

What is your Day 1?

You'll notice forty spaces next to *Cycle Day* on your chart, starting with 1. These represent each day of your cycle. Cycle length varies, so don't worry if you find you don't use all forty. And if your cycle length happens to be longer than forty days, use the extra charts included in your book to continue your tracking.

Cycle Day 1 is the first day you bleed. This means that you start using your chart on the first day of your period. If you've noticed that you spot bleed before your bleeding becomes more consistent, you'll still want to begin your chart with the first full day of bleeding, not a day of spotting only. If you're still feeling unsure of your Day 1, start your chart with the first day you find yourself reaching for a pad, tampon, menstrual cup, period underwear, or free-bleed pants.

STEP 2. Fill in the blank

Cycle Days. Now that you've figured out your Day 1, write the date of the month above Day 1. For example, if you notice that you have your first day of full bleeding (versus just spotting) on January 12, you'll write the number 12 above Cycle Day 1. On Cycle Day 2, you'll write 13, and so on.

Basal Body Temperature (BBT). You'll see two blank spaces next to the temperatures on the sides of your chart. This allows you to customize the chart to match your body. Some people are slightly warmer or cooler than others. These blank spaces allow you to write your baseline temperature. The *F/C* allows you to designate Fahrenheit or Celsius as a measurement. Begin to take your waking temperature (before you get out of bed) for a few days to decide what range your temperature tends to be. For example, you'll find out if you are generally 96–97°F, 97–98°F, 35–36°C, and so on.

You'll also see 0–9 listed vertically next to each of those blank lines. This makes it easy to mark daily BBT including the first decimal.

Category. Customize your tracking by writing in tracking categories of your choosing. Use your earlier work identifying your personal sensations to guide your category selection.

STEP 3. Fill in the bubble

To make tracking as simple and effective as possible, we use a fill-in-the-blank approach. Fill in the categories you want to track, and fill in the bubble when that tracking category is present on each cycle day.

Basal Body Temperature (BBT). On each day of your cycle, fill in the bubble that corresponds to the first decimal of the temperature on your thermometer.

Body Fluid. When you notice different types of body fluid present, fill in the bubble.

Category. When that category is present in your day, fill in the bubble.

Intensity. Rows 5 and 6 offer a 1-to-3 scale to rank your categories. To get the best visual of each category's rise and fall, follow these instructions:

If you rank the category as a one out of three, always fill in the bottom bubble.

If you rank the category as a two out of three, always fill in the bottom bubble and the middle bubble.

For a three out of three, fill in the bottom, middle, and top bubbles.

STEP 4. Beyond the bubble (optional)

Time of day. If you're noticing that a category is more or less present at a certain time of day, consider writing *AM* or *PM* on top of that day's bubble.

Luteinizing hormone (LH) or ovulation predictor kit (OPK) values. If you're using an ovulation predictor kit and gather values of LH daily, write that number on top of the day's bubble.

Color. If you're tracking the color of a body fluid, consider recording colors like brown, red, or pink by writing *B*, *R*, or *P* on that day's bubble.

Flow. Track the volume of your body fluids. You can track light, medium, or heavy by writing *L*, *M*, or *H* on that day's bubble.

Take a peek at a few other people's charts for inspiration:

Nasreen

Nasreen checks out her first tracking chart and immediately notices a few things—the ovulation predictor test strips she has been using don't seem to have the rise in numbers she was told to expect. She uses the test strips in the middle of her cycle as instructed by her provider, but she tests for a few extra days because she doesn't see any high numbers. She stops testing when the numbers go down, but she was surprised they didn't go higher. Nasreen is also surprised by some of her BBT tracking. She notices that her baseline temperature does not increase. Additionally, she has charted slippery fluid at multiple times during her cycle, all many days apart.

CYCLE

BASAL BODY TEMPERATURES

CYCLE DAY	1	2	3	4	5	6	7	8	9	10	11	12	13	14	15	16	17	18	19	20

Higher Baseline BBT — 36 F/C

Rows (9,8,7,6,5,4,3,2,1,0) with marked cells indicating temperatures.

Lower Baseline BBT — 35 F/C

BODY FLUIDS

CYCLE DAY	1	2	3	4	5	6	7	8	9	10	11	12	13	14	15	16	17	18	19	20
Bleeding	●	●	●	○	○	○	○	○	○	○	○	○	○	○	○	○	○	○	○	○
Spotting	○	○	○	●	○	○		○	○	○	○	○	○	○	○	○	○	○	○	○
Dry	○	○	○	○	○	○		○	○	○	○	○	○	○	○	○	○	○	○	○
Creamy	○	○	○	○	○	○	○	●	●	○	○	○	●	○	○	○	●	○	○	○
Slippery	○	○	○	○	○	○	○	○	○	●	○	○	○	○	●	○	○	●	○	●

CATEGORIES

	CYCLE DAY	1	2	3	4	5	6	7	8	9	10	11	12	13	14	15	16	17	18	19	20
1	Comfort	○	○	○	●	●	●	○	●	●	●	○	○	○	○	○	○	○	○	○	○
2	OPK	○	○	○	○	○	○	○	○	11	6	7	6	10	11	8	4	13	6	3	○
3		○	○	○	○	○	○	○	○	○	○	○	○	○	○	○	○	○	○	○	○
4		○	○	○	○	○	○	○	○	○	○	○	○	○	○	○	○	○	○	○	○
5		○	○	○	○	○	○	○	○	○	○	○	○	○	○	○	○	○	○	○	○
		○	○	○	○	○	○	○	○	○	○	○	○	○	○	○	○	○	○	○	○
6		○	○	○	○	○	○	○	○	○	○	○	○	○	○	○	○	○	○	○	○

NASREEN

BASAL BODY TEMPERATURES

CYCLE DAY	21	22	23	24	25	26	27	28	29	30	31	32	33	34	35	36	37	38	39	40

Higher Baseline BBT — **36** F/C (C circled)

Lower Baseline BBT — **35** F/C (C circled)

BODY FLUIDS

CYCLE DAY	21	22	23	24	25	26	27	28	29	30	31	32	33	34	35	36	37	38	39	40	
																					Bleeding
													●	●	●						Spotting
			●																		Dry
					●																Creamy
																					Slippery

CATEGORIES

CYCLE DAY	21	22	23	24	25	26	27	28	29	30	31	32	33	34	35	36	37	38	39	40		
																					Comfort	1
																					OPK	2
																						3
																						4
																						5
																						6

Ramona

Ramona finds that her charts seem to show a regular cyclical reflection of the shifts she notices in her mood and relationship to her work. In this particular chart, Ramona notices a day that seemed to be a bit of an outlier—Day 24. Ramona recalls that day and checks her calendar—she had been prepping for a show that day and had had an emotional talk with her sister at coffee. Ramona is surprised to see just how much those events impacted her day—it was a bit of a roller coaster.

CYCLE

MONTH _JAN_ DATE _12_ _13_ _14_ _15_ _16_ _17_ _18_ _19_ _20_ _21_ _22_ _23_ _24_ _25_ _26_ _27_ _28_ _29_ _30_ _31_

BASAL BODY TEMPERATURES

Higher Baseline BBT — 98 °F/°C

CYCLE DAY	1	2	3	4	5	6	7	8	9	10	11	12	13	14	15	16	17	18	19	20

(Grid of numbered bubbles 9 down to 0 for each cycle day)

Lower Baseline BBT — 97 °F/°C

(Grid of numbered bubbles 9 down to 0 for each cycle day)

BODY FLUIDS

CYCLE DAY	1	2	3	4	5	6	7	8	9	10	11	12	13	14	15	16	17	18	19	20
Bleeding	●	●	○	○	○	○	○	○	○	○	○	○	○	○	○	○	○	○	○	○
Spotting	○	○	●	●	●	○	○	○	○	○	○	○	○	○	○	○	○	○	○	○
Dry	○	○	○	○	○	●	○	○	○	○	○	○	○	○	○	○	○	○	○	○
Creamy	○	○	○	○	○	○	●	○	●	○	○	○	○	○	●	○	○	○	○	○
Slippery	○	○	○	○	○	○	○	○	●	○	●	○	●	○	○	○	○	○	○	○

CATEGORIES

	CYCLE DAY	1	2	3	4	5	6	7	8	9	10	11	12	13	14	15	16	17	18	19	20
1	Comfort	○	○	○	○	●	○	○	○	●	●	●	●	○	●	●	○	○	○	○	●
2	"ON"	●	●	○	●	○	●	●	○	●	●	●	●	●	●	●	○	●	○	○	○
3	"OFF"	○	○	○	○	○	○	○	●	○	○	○	○	○	○	○	○	○	●	●	○
4		○	○	○	○	○	○	○	○	○	○	○	○	○	○	○	○	○	○	○	○
5	SAD, HEAVY	○	○	○	○	○	○	○	○	○	○	○	○	○	○	○	●	○	●	○	○
6	LIGHT, CREATIVE	●	●	○	○	○	●	●	○	●	●	●	●	●	●	○	○	●	○	○	○

RAMONA

1 2 3 4 5 6 7 8 9 ___ ___ ___ ___ ___ ___ ___ ___ ___ ___ ___ ___   DATE FEB MONTH

| 21 | 22 | 23 | 24 | 25 | 26 | 27 | 28 | 29 | 30 | 31 | 32 | 33 | 34 | 35 | 36 | 37 | 38 | 39 | 40 | **CYCLE DAY** |

BASAL BODY TEMPERATURES

Higher Baseline BBT — 98 (F)/C

Lower Baseline BBT — 97 (F)/C

BODY FLUIDS

21	22	23	24	25	26	27	28	29	30	31	32	33	34	35	36	37	38	39	40	**CYCLE DAY**
																				Bleeding
																				Spotting
		●	●																	Dry
																				Creamy
																				Slippery

CATEGORIES

21	22	23	24	25	26	27	28	29	30	31	32	33	34	35	36	37	38	39	40	**CYCLE DAY**	
							●	●												Comfort	1
			●																	"ON"	2
	●	●	●	●		●		●												"OFF"	3
																					4
			●	●																	
●			●	●																	
●		●		●	●	●	●													SAD, HEAVY	5
		●																		
●			●																	LIGHT, CREATIVE	6

Mei

Mei looks at her chart and notices that although she had been worried that she wasn't feeling "enough" of many things in her relationship—arousal, desire, connection—she has clearly marked multiple phases of arousal and her personal signs of desire in her cycle. It seems these show up around the ovulatory phase and toward the end of the luteal phase right before her bleeding phase begins. What becomes clear to Mei is that she has assigned some sort of value to these categories without realizing it. Mei has been feeling like she needs the "right" amount of these to feel secure in her relationship. This no longer feels accurate to Mei, and she loosens up some of the pressure she had been putting on herself.

CYCLE

MONTH _AVG_   DATE _4 5 6 7 8 9 10 11 12 13 14 15 16 17 18 19 20 21 22 23_

BASAL BODY TEMPERATURES

Higher Baseline BBT — 97 F/C

CYCLE DAY	1	2	3	4	5	6	7	8	9	10	11	12	13	14	15	16	17	18	19	20
9																				●
8																				
7																			●	
6																				
5																●				
4				●																
3													●					●		
2		●														●				
1									●											
0	●				●															

Lower Baseline BBT — 96 F/C

CYCLE DAY	1	2	3	4	5	6	7	8	9	10	11	12	13	14	15	16	17	18	19	20
9		●																		
8								●												
7																				
6																				
5																				
4																				
3																				
2																				
1																				
0																				

BODY FLUIDS

CYCLE DAY	1	2	3	4	5	6	7	8	9	10	11	12	13	14	15	16	17	18	19	20
Bleeding	●	●	●	○	○	○	○	○	○	○	○	○	○	○	○	○	○	○	○	○
Spotting	○	○	○	○	○	○	○	○	○	○	○	○	○	○	○	○	○	○	○	○
Dry	○	○	○	○	○	○	○	○	○	○	○	○	○	○	○	○	○	○	○	○
Creamy	○	○	○	○	○	○	○	○	○	○	○	○	●	○	●	○	○	○	○	○
Slippery	○	○	○	○	○	○	○	○	○	○	○	○	○	○	○	○	●	●	●	○

CATEGORIES

	CYCLE DAY	1	2	3	4	5	6	7	8	9	10	11	12	13	14	15	16	17	18	19	20
1	Comfort	●	○	○	○	○	○	○	○	○	○	○	○	○	○	○	○	○	○	○	○
2	PIMPLES	○	○	○	○	○	○	○	○	○	○	○	○	○	○	○	○	○	○	○	○
3	BRIGHT MOOD	○	○	○	○	●	●	○	○	●	○	○	○	●	○	○	○	●	●	●	○
4	CRANKY MOOD	○	○	○	○	○	○	○	○	○	○	○	○	○	○	○	○	○	○	○	○
5	AROUSAL	○	○	○	○	○	○	○	○	○	○	○	○	○	○	○	○	●	●	●	●
		○	○	○	○	○	○	○	○	○	○	○	○	○	○	○	○	●	●	●	●
		○	○	○	○	○	○	○	○	○	○	○	○	○	○	○	○	●	●	●	●
6	FANTASIES	○	○	○	○	○	○	○	○	○	○	○	○	○	○	○	○	●	○	●	○
		○	○	○	○	○	○	○	○	○	○	○	○	○	○	○	○	●	○	●	○

24 25 26 27 28 29 30 31 1 2 3 4 5 __ __ __ __ __ __ DATE _SEPT_ MONTH

BASAL BODY TEMPERATURES

| 21 | 22 | 23 | 24 | 25 | 26 | 27 | 28 | 29 | 30 | 31 | 32 | 33 | 34 | 35 | 36 | 37 | 38 | 39 | 40 | CYCLE DAY |

Higher Baseline BBT

97 F C

Lower Baseline BBT

96 F C

BODY FLUIDS

| 21 | 22 | 23 | 24 | 25 | 26 | 27 | 28 | 29 | 30 | 31 | 32 | 33 | 34 | 35 | 36 | 37 | 38 | 39 | 40 | CYCLE DAY |

Bleeding
Spotting
Dry
Creamy
Slippery

CATEGORIES

| 21 | 22 | 23 | 24 | 25 | 26 | 27 | 28 | 29 | 30 | 31 | 32 | 33 | 34 | 35 | 36 | 37 | 38 | 39 | 40 | CYCLE DAY |

Comfort 1
PIMPLES 2
BRIGHT MOOD 3
CRANKY MOOD 4

AROUSAL 5

FANTASIES 6

Sam

Sam considers their chart at the end of their cycle. They feel truly proud of the progress they have made working toward a less painful relationship with their body and themself. They do notice two points in their chart where their self-critical thoughts seem higher. Sam notices that these coincide with two body fluid categories—bleeding and slippery. Sam wonders if they might have some discomfort with these body fluids and is curious about what they represent to them.

CYCLE

BASAL BODY TEMPERATURES

Higher Baseline BBT — 98 (F/C)

CYCLE DAY	1	2	3	4	5	6	7	8	9	10	11	12	13	14	15	16	17	18	19	20
9																				
8													●							
7															●		●	●		●
6												●							●	
5															●		●			
4						●														
3										●						●				
2				●																
1								●												
0	●	●																		

Lower Baseline BBT — 97 (F/C)

CYCLE DAY	1	2	3	4	5	6	7	8	9	10	11	12	13	14	15	16	17	18	19	20
9						●				●										
8																				
7		●		●				●												
6																				
5																				
4																				
3																				
2																				
1																				
0																				

BODY FLUIDS

CYCLE DAY	1	2	3	4	5	6	7	8	9	10	11	12	13	14	15	16	17	18	19	20
Bleeding	●	●	●																	
Spotting																				
Dry					●	●	●	●												
Creamy									●		●									
Slippery										●	●									

CATEGORIES

CYCLE DAY	1	2	3	4	5	6	7	8	9	10	11	12	13	14	15	16	17	18	19	20
1 Comfort					●	●	●	●												
2 RESPECT FOR BODY															●	●	●		●	
3 GOOD IN BODY						●	●										●			
4																				
5 SELF-CRITICISM										●	●									
	●									●	●									
	●			●																
6																				

19 20 21 22 _ _ _ _ _ _ _ _ _ _ _ _ _ _ _ _ _ DATE **NOV** MONTH

BASAL BODY TEMPERATURES

CYCLE DAY	21	22	23	24	25	26	27	28	29	30	31	32	33	34	35	36	37	38	39	40	

Higher Baseline BBT — 98 (F)/C

Marks: Day 21 filled "1"; Day 22 filled "3"; Day 23 filled "5"; Day 24 filled "3"

Lower Baseline BBT — 97 (F)/C

BODY FLUIDS

CYCLE DAY	21	22	23	24	25	26	27	28	29	30	31	32	33	34	35	36	37	38	39	40	
Bleeding	○	○	○	○	○	○	○	○	○	○	○	○	○	○	○	○	○	○	○	○	
Spotting	○	○	○	○	○	○	○	○	○	○	○	○	○	○	○	○	○	○	○	○	
Dry	○	●	●	●	○	○	○	○	○	○	○	○	○	○	○	○	○	○	○	○	
Creamy	○	○	○	○	○	○	○	○	○	○	○	○	○	○	○	○	○	○	○	○	
Slippery	○	○	○	○	○	○	○	○	○	○	○	○	○	○	○	○	○	○	○	○	

CATEGORIES

CYCLE DAY	21	22	23	24	25	26	27	28	29	30	31	32	33	34	35	36	37	38	39	40		
Comfort	○	○	●	○	○	○	○	○	○	○	○	○	○	○	○	○	○	○	○	○		1
RE-SPECT FOR BODY	○	●	●	○	○	○	○	○	○	○	○	○	○	○	○	○	○	○	○	○	○	2
GOOD IN BODY	●	●	○	○	○	○	○	○	○	○	○	○	○	○	○	○	○	○	○	○	○	3
	○	○	○	○	○	○	○	○	○	○	○	○	○	○	○	○	○	○	○	○		4
SELF-CRITICISM	○	○	○	○	○	○	○	○	○	○	○	○	○	○	○	○	○	○	○	○	○	5
	○	○	○	○	○	○	○	○	○	○	○	○	○	○	○	○	○	○	○	○		6

Ines

Ines looks at her chart. Just as expected, the bleeding phase of her cycle is accompanied by the most extreme of her endometriosis symptoms. Multiple days in a row she has severe pain and GI distress. What she wasn't expecting was the bit toward the end of her luteal phase—Ines has a pattern of increasing pain before she begins to bleed as well. Ines realizes that her window of pain reprieve is even shorter than she thought. This serves as a true motivation for her next provider visit.

CYCLE

MONTH _JUNE_ DATE 7 8 9 10 11 12 13 14 15 16 17 18 19 20 21 22 23 24 25 26

BASAL BODY TEMPERATURES

Higher Baseline BBT — 97 F/C

CYCLE DAY	1	2	3	4	5	6	7	8	9	10	11	12	13	14	15	16	17	18	19	20
9																				
8																				
7																				
6																				●
5																				
4																●				
3																				
2		●		●													●		●	
1										●	●									
0	●		●		●	●	●													

Lower Baseline BBT — 96 F/C

CYCLE DAY	1	2	3	4	5	6	7	8	9	10	11	12	13	14	15	16	17	18	19	20
9			●			●						●								
8		●						●					●							
7															●					
6																				
5																				
4																				
3																				
2																				
1																				
0																				

BODY FLUIDS

CYCLE DAY	1	2	3	4	5	6	7	8	9	10	11	12	13	14	15	16	17	18	19	20
Bleeding	●	●	●	●	●															
Spotting						●	●													
Dry																				
Creamy												●	●							
Slippery																	●	●		

CATEGORIES

	CYCLE DAY	1	2	3	4	5	6	7	8	9	10	11	12	13	14	15	16	17	18	19	20
1	Comfort						●									●	●		●		●
2	BLOATING	●	●	●	●	●	●	●													
3	VOMITING	●	●		●																
4																					
5	HOT, STABBING PAIN	●	●	●	●	●															
5	HOT, STABBING PAIN	●	●	●	●	●	●														
6	RADIATING PAIN	●	●	●																	
6	RADIATING PAIN	●	●	●		●		●	●		●										

INES

BASAL BODY TEMPERATURES

CYCLE DAY: 21 22 23 24 25 26 27 28 29 30 31 32 33 34 35 36 37 38 39 40

Higher Baseline BBT — 97 (F)/C

Filled values by cycle day: 21→2, 22→3, 23→4, 24→6, 25→6, 26→7, 27→5, 28→3, 29→5, 30→7, 31→4

Lower Baseline BBT — 96 (F)/C

BODY FLUIDS

CYCLE DAY: 21 22 23 24 25 26 27 28 29 30 31 32 33 34 35 36 37 38 39 40

Marker	Filled cycle days
Bleeding	
Spotting	
Dry	31
Creamy	22, 24
Slippery	

CATEGORIES

CYCLE DAY: 21 22 23 24 25 26 27 28 29 30 31 32 33 34 35 36 37 38 39 40

Category	Filled cycle days
Comfort — 1	21, 22
BLOATING — 2	23, 24, 26, 27, 28, 29, 30, 31
VOMITING — 3	
4	
HOT, STABBING PAIN — 5	
RADIATING PAIN — 6	26, 29, 30, 31

Georgia

Georgia sees on paper what she had already been feeling—the week to ten days leading up to her bleeding phase felt like she was all over the place. Her attention felt scattered, her anxiety was higher, and the mornings with getting the kids out the door were chaos. Georgia did notice two days that seemed a bit confusing and difficult to interpret—Days 2 and 8. She examines her chart and is a bit baffled as she has filled in the bubbles for chaotic a.m. as well as good focus and attention on those days. She takes out her calendar to cross-reference. Oh. It snowed on Days 2 and 8! All three of her kids refused their snowsuits, major tantrums were had, and every drop-off was late. Georgia realized that the shift she noticed was environmental due to the snow and not hormonal.

CYCLE

MONTH FEB   DATE 14 15 16 17 18 19 20 21 22 23 24 25 26 27 28 29 1 2 3 4

BASAL BODY TEMPERATURES

Higher Baseline BBT — 37 °C

CYCLE DAY	1	2	3	4	5	6	7	8	9	10	11	12	13	14	15	16	17	18	19	20
9																				
8																				
7																				
6																				
5																	●			
4												●							●	
3													●		●					
2						●										●				●
1				●			●													
0	●	●	●							●										

Lower Baseline BBT — 36 °C

CYCLE DAY	1	2	3	4	5	6	7	8	9	10	11	12	13	14	15	16	17	18	19	20
9		●			●					●										
8																				
7–0																				

BODY FLUIDS

CYCLE DAY	1	2	3	4	5	6	7	8	9	10	11	12	13	14	15	16	17	18	19	20
Bleeding	●	●	●																	
Spotting				●		●														
Dry																				
Creamy							●	●	●											
Slippery												●								

CATEGORIES

	CYCLE DAY	1	2	3	4	5	6	7	8	9	10	11	12	13	14	15	16	17	18	19	20
1	Comfort	●			●							●	●		●						
2	SEX						●													●	
3	CHAOTIC AM		●						●												
4																					
5	CLEAR THOUGHTS			●	●	●	●	●	●	●	●										
6	FOCUS ON KIDS	●	●	●		●	●	●	●												

GEORGIA

5 6 7 8 9 10 11 12 _____

BASAL BODY TEMPERATURES

CYCLE DAY	21	22	23	24	25	26	27	28	29	30	31	32	33	34	35	36	37	38	39	40

Higher Baseline BBT — 37 F/**C**

Temperature grid digits 9 through 0. Filled marks:
- Day 22: 2 filled
- Day 23: 1 filled
- Day 24: 2 filled
- Day 25: 1 filled
- Day 26: 2, 1 filled
- Day 28: 3 filled
- Day 21: 0 filled, 1 filled

Lower Baseline BBT — 36 F/**C**

BODY FLUIDS

CYCLE DAY	21	22	23	24	25	26	27	28	29	30	31	32	33	34	35	36	37	38	39	40	
	○	○	○	○	○	○	○	○	○	○	○	○	○	○	○	○	○	○	○	○	Bleeding
	○	○	○	○	○	○	○	○	○	○	○	○	○	○	○	○	○	○	○	○	Spotting
	○	○	○	○	○	○	○	○	○	○	○	○	○	○	○	○	○	○	○	○	Dry
	○	○	●	○	○	○	○	○	○	○	○	○	○	○	○	○	○	○	○	○	Creamy
	○	○	○	○	○	○	○	○	○	○	○	○	○	○	○	○	○	○	○	○	Slippery

CATEGORIES

CYCLE DAY	21	22	23	24	25	26	27	28	29	30	31	32	33	34	35	36	37	38	39	40		
	○	○	○	○	○	○	○	○	○	○	○	○	○	○	○	○	○	○	○	○	Comfort	1
	○	○	○	○	○	○	○	●	○	○	○	○	○	○	○	○	○	○	○	○	SEX	2
	●	●	●	●	●	●	●	●	○	○	○	○	○	○	○	○	○	○	○	○	CHAOTIC AM	3
	○	○	○	○	○	○	○	○	○	○	○	○	○	○	○	○	○	○	○	○		4
	○	○	○	○	○	○	○	○	○	○	○	○	○	○	○	○	○	○	○	○		
	●	○	○	○	○	○	○	○	○	○	○	○	○	○	○	○	○	○	○	○	CLEAR THOUGHTS	5
	○	○	○	○	○	○	○	○	○	○	○	○	○	○	○	○	○	○	○	○		
	●	○	○	○	○	○	○	○	○	○	○	○	○	○	○	○	○	○	○	○		
	●	●	○	○	○	○	○	○	○	○	○	○	○	○	○	○	○	○	○	○	FOCUS ON KIDS	6

Talia

Tracking has been a bit more intense this last cycle, as Talia has been prepping for a more targeted pain intervention. She wants to have a solid foundation of understanding her cycle and patterns as she gets into her pelvic pain treatment plan. As she reviews her chart, she sees a clear pattern. Every time after she spends more than a few days with her girlfriend, she has an increased trauma response. Talia understands that this pattern has nothing to do with her hormones.

CYCLE

MONTH _SEPT_ DATE _9_ _10_ _11_ _12_ _13_ _14_ _15_ _16_ _17_ _18_ _19_ _20_ _21_ _22_ _23_ _24_ _25_ _26_ _27_ _28_

BASAL BODY TEMPERATURES

Higher Baseline BBT — 98 (F)/C

Lower Baseline BBT — 97 (F)/C

CYCLE DAY: 1 2 3 4 5 6 7 8 9 10 11 12 13 14 15 16 17 18 19 20

BODY FLUIDS

CYCLE DAY	1	2	3	4	5	6	7	8	9	10	11	12	13	14	15	16	17	18	19	20
Bleeding	●	●	●	●	○	○	○	○	○	○	○	○	○	○	○	○	○	○	○	○
Spotting	○	○	○	○	●	●	●	○	○	○	○	○	○	○	○	○	○	○	○	○
Dry	○	○	○	○	○	○	○	○	○	○	○	○	○	○	○	○	○	○	○	○
Creamy	○	○	○	○	○	○	○	○	○	○	○	○	○	○	○	○	○	○	○	○
Slippery	○	○	○	○	○	○	○	○	○	○	○	○	○	●	●	●	○	○	○	○

CATEGORIES

	CYCLE DAY	1	2	3	4	5	6	7	8	9	10	11	12	13	14	15	16	17	18	19	20
1	Comfort	●	●	○	○	●	●	●	○	○	●	●	○	●	●	●	●	●	○	○	○
2	CRAMPING	●	○	○	○	○	○	○	○	○	○	○	○	○	○	○	○	○	○	○	○
3	GROUNDED, SAFE	●	○	○	○	●	●	●	○	○	●	●	●	●	●	○	●	●	●	●	○
4	SEE GF	○	●	●	●	○	●	●	●	●	○	●	○	●	○	●	●	●	○	●	●
5	NUMB	○	○	○	○	○	○	○	○	●	○	○	○	○	○	○	○	○	○	○	○
		○	○	○	○	○	○	○	●	●	○	○	○	○	○	○	○	○	○	○	○
6	HOLLOW	○	○	○	●	○	○	○	●	●	○	○	○	○	●	○	○	○	○	○	○

TALIA

BASAL BODY TEMPERATURES

CYCLE DAY 21 22 23 24 25 26 27 28 29 30 31 32 33 34 35 36 37 38 39 40

Higher Baseline BBT — 98 (F)/C

Lower Baseline BBT — 97 (F)/C

BODY FLUIDS

CYCLE DAY 21 22 23 24 25 26 27 28 29 30 31 32 33 34 35 36 37 38 39 40

- Bleeding
- Spotting
- Dry
- Creamy
- Slippery

CATEGORIES

CYCLE DAY 21 22 23 24 25 26 27 28 29 30 31 32 33 34 35 36 37 38 39 40

Comfort	1
CRAMPING	2
GROUNDED, SAFE	3
SEE GF	4
NUMB	5
HOLLOW	6

Aisha

Aisha glances at her first tracking chart. First, her cycle is shorter than she thought. Second, there is a clear hormonal link to the tough anxiety and paranoia she has been feeling about work. She also notices that her temperatures don't stay high in the latter half of her cycle. Aisha's panic and jittery dread show up on her chart in the five to seven days before her bleeding phase begins.

CYCLE

BASAL BODY TEMPERATURES

Higher Baseline BBT — 98 F/C

CYCLE DAY	1	2	3	4	5	6	7	8	9	10	11	12	13	14	15	16	17	18	19	20
9	9	9	9	9	9	9	9	9	9	9	9	9	9	9	9	9	9	9	9	9
8	8	8	8	8	8	8	8	8	8	8	8	8	8	8	8	8	8	8	8	8
7	7	7	7	7	7	7	7	7	7	7	7	7	7	7	7	7	7	7	7	7
6	6	6	6	6	6	6	6	6	6	6	6	6	6	6	6	6	6	6	6	6
5	5	5	5	5	5	5	5	5	5	5	5	5	5	5	5	●	5	5	5	5
4	4	4	4	4	4	4	4	4	4	4	4	4	4	●	4	4	4	4	4	4
3	3	3	3	3	●	3	3	3	3	3	3	3	3	●	3	3	3	3	3	3
2	2	2	2	2	2	2	2	2	2	2	2	2	●	2	2	2	2	2	●	2
1	1	1	1	1	1	1	1	1	●	1	1	1	●	1	1	1	1	1	1	●
●	0	0	0	0	0	0	0	0	0	●	0	0	0	0	0	0	0	0	0	0

Lower Baseline BBT — 97 F/C

CYCLE DAY	1	2	3	4	5	6	7	8	9	10	11	12	13	14	15	16	17	18	19	20
9	9	9	●	9	9	●	9	9	9	9	9	●	9	9	9	9	9	9	9	9
8	8	●	8	8	8	8	8	●	8	8	8	8	8	8	8	8	8	8	8	8
7	●	7	7	7	7	7	7	7	7	7	7	7	●	7	7	7	7	7	7	7
6	6	6	6	6	6	6	6	6	6	6	6	6	6	6	6	6	6	6	6	6
5	5	5	5	●	5	5	5	5	5	5	5	5	5	5	5	5	5	5	5	5
4	4	4	4	4	4	4	4	4	4	4	4	4	4	4	4	4	4	4	4	4
3	3	3	3	3	3	3	3	3	3	3	3	3	3	3	3	3	3	3	3	3
2	2	2	2	2	2	2	2	2	2	2	2	2	2	2	2	2	2	2	2	2
1	1	1	1	1	1	1	1	1	1	1	1	1	1	1	1	1	1	1	1	1
0	0	0	0	0	0	0	0	0	0	0	0	0	0	0	0	0	0	0	0	0

BODY FLUIDS

CYCLE DAY	1	2	3	4	5	6	7	8	9	10	11	12	13	14	15	16	17	18	19	20
Bleeding	●	●	●	●	○	○	○	○	○	○	○	○	○	○	○	○	○	○	○	○
Spotting	○	○	○	○	○	○	○	○	○	○	○	○	○	○	○	○	○	○	○	○
Dry	○	○	○	○	○	○	○	○	○	○	○	○	○	○	○	○	○	○	○	○
Creamy	○	○	○	○	○	○	○	○	○	●	●	○	○	○	○	○	○	○	●	○
Slippery	○	○	○	○	○	○	○	○	○	○	○	○	●	○	●	○	○	○	○	○

CATEGORIES

CYCLE DAY	1	2	3	4	5	6	7	8	9	10	11	12	13	14	15	16	17	18	19	20
1 Comfort	○	●	●	●	○	●	○	○	●	○	○	●	●	●	○	○	○	○	○	○
2 STOMACH DROPS PANIC	○	○	○	○	○	○	○	○	○	○	○	○	○	○	○	○	○	○	○	○
3 FIXATION ON JOB	●	○	○	○	○	○	○	○	○	○	○	○	○	○	●	●	○	○	●	○
4	○	○	○	○	○	○	○	○	○	○	○	○	○	○	○	○	○	○	○	○
	○	○	○	○	○	○	○	○	○	○	○	○	○	○	○	○	○	○	○	●
5 JITTERY ANXIETY	○	○	○	○	○	○	○	○	○	○	○	○	○	○	○	○	○	○	○	●
	○	●	○	○	○	○	○	○	○	○	○	○	○	○	○	○	○	○	○	○
MENTAL	○	●	○	○	○	○	○	○	○	○	○	○	○	○	○	○	○	○	○	○
6 EXHAUSTION	●	●	○	○	○	○	○	○	○	○	○	○	○	○	○	○	○	○	○	○

21 22 23 24 25 26 _ _ _ _ _ _ _ _ _ _ _ _ _ _ _ _ _ _ DATE **DEC** MONTH

BASAL BODY TEMPERATURES

CYCLE DAY	21	22	23	24	25	26	27	28	29	30	31	32	33	34	35	36	37	38	39	40

Higher Baseline BBT — 98 (F)C

Lower Baseline BBT — 97 (F)C

BODY FLUIDS

CYCLE DAY	21	22	23	24	25	26	27	28	29	30	31	32	33	34	35	36	37	38	39	40	
Bleeding																					
Spotting																					
Dry		●		●																	
Creamy																					
Slippery																					

CATEGORIES

CYCLE DAY	21	22	23	24	25	26	27	28	29	30	31	32	33	34	35	36	37	38	39	40	
Comfort 1																					
STOMACH DROPS PANIC 2			●		●	●															
FIXATION ON JOB 3		●	●		●	●															
4																					
			●		●	●															
			●	●	●	●															
JITTERY ANXIETY 5	●		●	●	●	●															
MENTAL EXHAUSTION 6		●																			

12.

Tracking Charts

In the pursuit of knowing your own body, this chapter is all yours.

After each tracking chart, you will find a guide to help identify what went well with your most recent cycle and what you might want to refine going into the next.

Track your hormones and change your life.

CYCLE

MONTH _____ DATE ____ ____ ____ ____ ____ ____ ____ ____ ____ ____ ____ ____ ____

BASAL BODY TEMPERATURES

CYCLE DAY 1 2 3 4 5 6 7 8 9 10 11 12 13 14 15 16 17 18 19 20

_____ F/C — Higher Baseline BBT

Values per day: 9 8 7 6 5 4 3 2 1 0

_____ F/C — Lower Baseline BBT

Values per day: 9 8 7 6 5 4 3 2 1 0

BODY FLUIDS

CYCLE DAY 1 2 3 4 5 6 7 8 9 10 11 12 13 14 15 16 17 18 19 20

Bleeding	O	O	O	O	O	O	O	O	O	O	O	O	O	O	O	O	O	O	O	O
Spotting	O	O	O	O	O	O	O	O	O	O	O	O	O	O	O	O	O	O	O	O
Dry	O	O	O	O	O	O	O	O	O	O	O	O	O	O	O	O	O	O	O	O
Creamy	O	O	O	O	O	O	O	O	O	O	O	O	O	O	O	O	O	O	O	O
Slippery	O	O	O	O	O	O	O	O	O	O	O	O	O	O	O	O	O	O	O	O

CATEGORIES

CYCLE DAY 1 2 3 4 5 6 7 8 9 10 11 12 13 14 15 16 17 18 19 20

1 Comfort

2

3

4

5

6

BASAL BODY TEMPERATURES

| CYCLE DAY | 21 | 22 | 23 | 24 | 25 | 26 | 27 | 28 | 29 | 30 | 31 | 32 | 33 | 34 | 35 | 36 | 37 | 38 | 39 | 40 |

Higher Baseline BBT — _____ F/C

Digits 9 through 0 (rows for each temperature value)

Lower Baseline BBT — _____ F/C

Digits 9 through 0 (rows for each temperature value)

BODY FLUIDS

CYCLE DAY	21	22	23	24	25	26	27	28	29	30	31	32	33	34	35	36	37	38	39	40	
	O	O	O	O	O	O	O	O	O	O	O	O	O	O	O	O	O	O	O	O	Bleeding
	O	O	O	O	O	O	O	O	O	O	O	O	O	O	O	O	O	O	O	O	Spotting
	O	O	O	O	O	O	O	O	O	O	O	O	O	O	O	O	O	O	O	O	Dry
	O	O	O	O	O	O	O	O	O	O	O	O	O	O	O	O	O	O	O	O	Creamy
	O	O	O	O	O	O	O	O	O	O	O	O	O	O	O	O	O	O	O	O	Slippery

CATEGORIES

CYCLE DAY	21	22	23	24	25	26	27	28	29	30	31	32	33	34	35	36	37	38	39	40		
	O	O	O	O	O	O	O	O	O	O	O	O	O	O	O	O	O	O	O	O	Comfort	1
	O	O	O	O	O	O	O	O	O	O	O	O	O	O	O	O	O	O	O	O		2
	O	O	O	O	O	O	O	O	O	O	O	O	O	O	O	O	O	O	O	O		3
	O	O	O	O	O	O	O	O	O	O	O	O	O	O	O	O	O	O	O	O		4
	O	O	O	O	O	O	O	O	O	O	O	O	O	O	O	O	O	O	O	O		
	O	O	O	O	O	O	O	O	O	O	O	O	O	O	O	O	O	O	O	O		
	O	O	O	O	O	O	O	O	O	O	O	O	O	O	O	O	O	O	O	O		5
	O	O	O	O	O	O	O	O	O	O	O	O	O	O	O	O	O	O	O	O		
	O	O	O	O	O	O	O	O	O	O	O	O	O	O	O	O	O	O	O	O		
	O	O	O	O	O	O	O	O	O	O	O	O	O	O	O	O	O	O	O	O		6

CYCLE REVIEW

Analyze your last cycle and prepare for your next

BASELINE INSIGHTS

BASAL BODY TEMPERATURE

Can you identify a significant and sustained temperature increase and the day it began?   ○ Yes   ○ No   ○ I'm not sure

_____

_____

BODY FLUID

Can you identify which day you experienced the most slippery fluid for this last cycle?   ○ Yes   ○ No   ○ I'm not sure

_____

_____

Could you easily differentiate bleeding and spotting for this last cycle?   ○ Yes   ○ No   ○ I'm not sure

_____

_____

Did you notice other body fluids during this last cycle?   ○ Yes   ○ No   ○ I'm not sure

_____

_____

PATTERNS

Starting with comfort, *review your list of categories tracked last cycle.*

Were you able to identify feelings of *comfort* during your last cycle?   ○ Yes   ○ No   ○ I'm not sure

Did you notice a change in how you felt on the days when comfort was present?   ○ Yes   ○ No   ○ I'm not sure

Write your other categories from last cycle below and use symbols for "More," "Less," and "I'm not sure."

(+) More   (−) Less   (?) I'm not sure

Are categories more or less present during the bleeding phase of your cycle?

____○____ ____○____ ____○____ ____○____ ____○

What categories seem to be more or less present when you notice slippery cervical fluid?

____○____ ____○____ ____○____ ____○____ ____○

What categories seem to be more or less present right before your next bleeding phase?

____○____ ____○____ ____○____ ____○____ ____○

GENERAL MOOD

Are you getting what you need out of tracking?

○ Yes, this is totally working   ○ I think I'm onto something   ○ Not yet, finding more support feels like a good next step

What patterns are you curious about for your next cycle?

_____

Which categories appear unrelated to phases of your cycle?

_____

CATEGORY INSIGHTS

Write your categories from last cycle below and use symbols for keeping, refining, and dropping those descriptions.

Do any categories need a bit of refining?   What categories are you going to track next cycle?

(✔) Keep   (→) Refine   (✗) Drop

	○	
	○	
	○	
	○	
	○	

CYCLE PREVIEW

What are your 3 goals for this next cycle of tracking?

_____   _____   _____

What will you do differently for your next cycle?

_____

_____

What are 2 ways you can introduce comfort, safety, and/or pleasure into your cycle?

_____   _____

What are 2 ways you can make cycle tracking easier for you?

_____   _____

CYCLE

MONTH _____ DATE _____

BASAL BODY TEMPERATURES

CYCLE DAY	1	2	3	4	5	6	7	8	9	10	11	12	13	14	15	16	17	18	19	20

_____ F/C — Higher Baseline BBT

Values 9, 8, 7, 6, 5, 4, 3, 2, 1, 0 (each as selectable bubbles for every cycle day)

_____ F/C — Lower Baseline BBT

Values 9, 8, 7, 6, 5, 4, 3, 2, 1, 0 (each as selectable bubbles for every cycle day)

BODY FLUIDS

CYCLE DAY	1	2	3	4	5	6	7	8	9	10	11	12	13	14	15	16	17	18	19	20
Bleeding	O	O	O	O	O	O	O	O	O	O	O	O	O	O	O	O	O	O	O	O
Spotting	O	O	O	O	O	O	O	O	O	O	O	O	O	O	O	O	O	O	O	O
Dry	O	O	O	O	O	O	O	O	O	O	O	O	O	O	O	O	O	O	O	O
Creamy	O	O	O	O	O	O	O	O	O	O	O	O	O	O	O	O	O	O	O	O
Slippery	O	O	O	O	O	O	O	O	O	O	O	O	O	O	O	O	O	O	O	O

CATEGORIES

CYCLE DAY	1	2	3	4	5	6	7	8	9	10	11	12	13	14	15	16	17	18	19	20
1 Comfort	O	O	O	O	O	O	O	O	O	O	O	O	O	O	O	O	O	O	O	O
2	O	O	O	O	O	O	O	O	O	O	O	O	O	O	O	O	O	O	O	O
3	O	O	O	O	O	O	O	O	O	O	O	O	O	O	O	O	O	O	O	O
4	O	O	O	O	O	O	O	O	O	O	O	O	O	O	O	O	O	O	O	O
5	O	O	O	O	O	O	O	O	O	O	O	O	O	O	O	O	O	O	O	O
5	O	O	O	O	O	O	O	O	O	O	O	O	O	O	O	O	O	O	O	O
5	O	O	O	O	O	O	O	O	O	O	O	O	O	O	O	O	O	O	O	O
6	O	O	O	O	O	O	O	O	O	O	O	O	O	O	O	O	O	O	O	O
6	O	O	O	O	O	O	O	O	O	O	O	O	O	O	O	O	O	O	O	O
6	O	O	O	O	O	O	O	O	O	O	O	O	O	O	O	O	O	O	O	O

BASAL BODY TEMPERATURES

| 21 | 22 | 23 | 24 | 25 | 26 | 27 | 28 | 29 | 30 | 31 | 32 | 33 | 34 | 35 | 36 | 37 | 38 | 39 | 40 | **CYCLE DAY** |

Higher Baseline BBT — _____ F/C

Rows (top to bottom): 9 8 7 6 5 4 3 2 1 0 (each repeated across all cycle day columns)

Lower Baseline BBT — _____ F/C

Rows (top to bottom): 9 8 7 6 5 4 3 2 1 0 (each repeated across all cycle day columns)

BODY FLUIDS

21	22	23	24	25	26	27	28	29	30	31	32	33	34	35	36	37	38	39	40	**CYCLE DAY**
○	○	○	○	○	○	○	○	○	○	○	○	○	○	○	○	○	○	○	○	Bleeding
○	○	○	○	○	○	○	○	○	○	○	○	○	○	○	○	○	○	○	○	Spotting
○	○	○	○	○	○	○	○	○	○	○	○	○	○	○	○	○	○	○	○	Dry
○	○	○	○	○	○	○	○	○	○	○	○	○	○	○	○	○	○	○	○	Creamy
○	○	○	○	○	○	○	○	○	○	○	○	○	○	○	○	○	○	○	○	Slippery

CATEGORIES

21	22	23	24	25	26	27	28	29	30	31	32	33	34	35	36	37	38	39	40	**CYCLE DAY**	
○	○	○	○	○	○	○	○	○	○	○	○	○	○	○	○	○	○	○	○	Comfort	1
○	○	○	○	○	○	○	○	○	○	○	○	○	○	○	○	○	○	○	○		2
○	○	○	○	○	○	○	○	○	○	○	○	○	○	○	○	○	○	○	○		3
○	○	○	○	○	○	○	○	○	○	○	○	○	○	○	○	○	○	○	○		4
○	○	○	○	○	○	○	○	○	○	○	○	○	○	○	○	○	○	○	○		
○	○	○	○	○	○	○	○	○	○	○	○	○	○	○	○	○	○	○	○		
○	○	○	○	○	○	○	○	○	○	○	○	○	○	○	○	○	○	○	○		5
○	○	○	○	○	○	○	○	○	○	○	○	○	○	○	○	○	○	○	○		
○	○	○	○	○	○	○	○	○	○	○	○	○	○	○	○	○	○	○	○		
○	○	○	○	○	○	○	○	○	○	○	○	○	○	○	○	○	○	○	○		6

CYCLE REVIEW

Analyze your last cycle and prepare for your next

BASELINE INSIGHTS

BASAL BODY TEMPERATURE

Can you identify a significant and sustained temperature increase and the day it began? ○ Yes ○ No ○ I'm not sure

_____

_____

BODY FLUID

Can you identify which day you experienced the most slippery fluid for this last cycle?   ○ Yes ○ No ○ I'm not sure

_____

_____

Could you easily differentiate bleeding and spotting for this last cycle?   ○ Yes ○ No ○ I'm not sure

_____

_____

Did you notice other body fluids during this last cycle?   ○ Yes ○ No ○ I'm not sure

_____

_____

PATTERNS

Starting with **comfort,** *review your list of categories tracked last cycle.*

Were you able to identify feelings of *comfort* during your last cycle?   ○ Yes ○ No ○ I'm not sure

Did you notice a change in how you felt on the days when comfort was present?   ○ Yes ○ No ○ I'm not sure

Write your other categories from last cycle below and use symbols for "More," "Less," and "I'm not sure."

(+) More   (−) Less   (?) I'm not sure

Are categories more or less present during the bleeding phase of your cycle?

____○____ ____○____ ____○____ ____○____ ____○

What categories seem to be more or less present when you notice slippery cervical fluid?

____○____ ____○____ ____○____ ____○____ ____○

What categories seem to be more or less present right before your next bleeding phase?

____○____ ____○____ ____○____ ____○____ ____○

GENERAL MOOD

Are you getting what you need out of tracking?

○ Yes, this is totally working   ○ I think I'm onto something   ○ Not yet, finding more support feels like a good next step

What patterns are you curious about for your next cycle?

_____

Which categories appear unrelated to phases of your cycle?

_____

CATEGORY INSIGHTS

Write your categories from last cycle below and use symbols for keeping, refining, and dropping those descriptions.

Do any categories need a bit of refining?   What categories are you going to track next cycle?

(✔) Keep   (→) Refine   (✗) Drop

_____ ○ _____

_____ ○ _____

_____ ○ _____

_____ ○ _____

_____ ○ _____

CYCLE PREVIEW

What are your 3 goals for this next cycle of tracking?

_____   _____   _____

What will you do differently for your next cycle?

_____

_____

What are 2 ways you can introduce comfort, safety, and/or pleasure into your cycle?

_____   _____

What are 2 ways you can make cycle tracking easier for you?

_____   _____

CYCLE

MONTH _____ DATE ___ __ __ __ __ __ __ __ __ __ __ __ __ __

BASAL BODY TEMPERATURES

Higher Baseline BBT _____ F/C

CYCLE DAY	1	2	3	4	5	6	7	8	9	10	11	12	13	14	15	16	17	18	19	20
	9	9	9	9	9	9	9	9	9	9	9	9	9	9	9	9	9	9	9	9
	8	8	8	8	8	8	8	8	8	8	8	8	8	8	8	8	8	8	8	8
	7	7	7	7	7	7	7	7	7	7	7	7	7	7	7	7	7	7	7	7
	6	6	6	6	6	6	6	6	6	6	6	6	6	6	6	6	6	6	6	6
	5	5	5	5	5	5	5	5	5	5	5	5	5	5	5	5	5	5	5	5
	4	4	4	4	4	4	4	4	4	4	4	4	4	4	4	4	4	4	4	4
	3	3	3	3	3	3	3	3	3	3	3	3	3	3	3	3	3	3	3	3
	2	2	2	2	2	2	2	2	2	2	2	2	2	2	2	2	2	2	2	2
	1	1	1	1	1	1	1	1	1	1	1	1	1	1	1	1	1	1	1	1
	0	0	0	0	0	0	0	0	0	0	0	0	0	0	0	0	0	0	0	0

Lower Baseline BBT _____ F/C

	9	9	9	9	9	9	9	9	9	9	9	9	9	9	9	9	9	9	9	9
	8	8	8	8	8	8	8	8	8	8	8	8	8	8	8	8	8	8	8	8
	7	7	7	7	7	7	7	7	7	7	7	7	7	7	7	7	7	7	7	7
	6	6	6	6	6	6	6	6	6	6	6	6	6	6	6	6	6	6	6	6
	5	5	5	5	5	5	5	5	5	5	5	5	5	5	5	5	5	5	5	5
	4	4	4	4	4	4	4	4	4	4	4	4	4	4	4	4	4	4	4	4
	3	3	3	3	3	3	3	3	3	3	3	3	3	3	3	3	3	3	3	3
	2	2	2	2	2	2	2	2	2	2	2	2	2	2	2	2	2	2	2	2
	1	1	1	1	1	1	1	1	1	1	1	1	1	1	1	1	1	1	1	1
	0	0	0	0	0	0	0	0	0	0	0	0	0	0	0	0	0	0	0	0

BODY FLUIDS

CYCLE DAY	1	2	3	4	5	6	7	8	9	10	11	12	13	14	15	16	17	18	19	20
Bleeding	O	O	O	O	O	O	O	O	O	O	O	O	O	O	O	O	O	O	O	O
Spotting	O	O	O	O	O	O	O	O	O	O	O	O	O	O	O	O	O	O	O	O
Dry	O	O	O	O	O	O	O	O	O	O	O	O	O	O	O	O	O	O	O	O
Creamy	O	O	O	O	O	O	O	O	O	O	O	O	O	O	O	O	O	O	O	O
Slippery	O	O	O	O	O	O	O	O	O	O	O	O	O	O	O	O	O	O	O	O

CATEGORIES

CYCLE DAY	1	2	3	4	5	6	7	8	9	10	11	12	13	14	15	16	17	18	19	20
1 Comfort	O	O	O	O	O	O	O	O	O	O	O	O	O	O	O	O	O	O	O	O
2	O	O	O	O	O	O	O	O	O	O	O	O	O	O	O	O	O	O	O	O
3	O	O	O	O	O	O	O	O	O	O	O	O	O	O	O	O	O	O	O	O
4	O	O	O	O	O	O	O	O	O	O	O	O	O	O	O	O	O	O	O	O
5	O	O	O	O	O	O	O	O	O	O	O	O	O	O	O	O	O	O	O	O
	O	O	O	O	O	O	O	O	O	O	O	O	O	O	O	O	O	O	O	O
	O	O	O	O	O	O	O	O	O	O	O	O	O	O	O	O	O	O	O	O
6	O	O	O	O	O	O	O	O	O	O	O	O	O	O	O	O	O	O	O	O
	O	O	O	O	O	O	O	O	O	O	O	O	O	O	O	O	O	O	O	O
	O	O	O	O	O	O	O	O	O	O	O	O	O	O	O	O	O	O	O	O

BASAL BODY TEMPERATURES

| | 21 | 22 | 23 | 24 | 25 | 26 | 27 | 28 | 29 | 30 | 31 | 32 | 33 | 34 | 35 | 36 | 37 | 38 | 39 | 40 | CYCLE DAY |

Higher Baseline BBT — values 9 8 7 6 5 4 3 2 1 0 for each cycle day 21–40

_____ F/C

Lower Baseline BBT — values 9 8 7 6 5 4 3 2 1 0 for each cycle day 21–40

_____ F/C

BODY FLUIDS

	21	22	23	24	25	26	27	28	29	30	31	32	33	34	35	36	37	38	39	40	CYCLE DAY
	O	O	O	O	O	O	O	O	O	O	O	O	O	O	O	O	O	O	O	O	Bleeding
	O	O	O	O	O	O	O	O	O	O	O	O	O	O	O	O	O	O	O	O	Spotting
	O	O	O	O	O	O	O	O	O	O	O	O	O	O	O	O	O	O	O	O	Dry
	O	O	O	O	O	O	O	O	O	O	O	O	O	O	O	O	O	O	O	O	Creamy
	O	O	O	O	O	O	O	O	O	O	O	O	O	O	O	O	O	O	O	O	Slippery

CATEGORIES

	21	22	23	24	25	26	27	28	29	30	31	32	33	34	35	36	37	38	39	40	CYCLE DAY	
	O	O	O	O	O	O	O	O	O	O	O	O	O	O	O	O	O	O	O	O	Comfort	1
	O	O	O	O	O	O	O	O	O	O	O	O	O	O	O	O	O	O	O	O		2
	O	O	O	O	O	O	O	O	O	O	O	O	O	O	O	O	O	O	O	O		3
	O	O	O	O	O	O	O	O	O	O	O	O	O	O	O	O	O	O	O	O		4
	O	O	O	O	O	O	O	O	O	O	O	O	O	O	O	O	O	O	O	O		
	O	O	O	O	O	O	O	O	O	O	O	O	O	O	O	O	O	O	O	O		5
	O	O	O	O	O	O	O	O	O	O	O	O	O	O	O	O	O	O	O	O		
	O	O	O	O	O	O	O	O	O	O	O	O	O	O	O	O	O	O	O	O		
	O	O	O	O	O	O	O	O	O	O	O	O	O	O	O	O	O	O	O	O		6

CYCLE REVIEW

Analyze your last cycle and prepare for your next

BASELINE INSIGHTS

BASAL BODY TEMPERATURE

Can you identify a significant and sustained temperature increase and the day it began? ○ Yes ○ No ○ I'm not sure

_____

_____

BODY FLUID

Can you identify which day you experienced the most slippery fluid for this last cycle? ○ Yes ○ No ○ I'm not sure

_____

_____

Could you easily differentiate bleeding and spotting for this last cycle? ○ Yes ○ No ○ I'm not sure

_____

_____

Did you notice other body fluids during this last cycle? ○ Yes ○ No ○ I'm not sure

_____

_____

PATTERNS

Starting with comfort, review your list of categories tracked last cycle.

Were you able to identify feelings of *comfort* during your last cycle? ○ Yes ○ No ○ I'm not sure

Did you notice a change in how you felt on the days when comfort was present? ○ Yes ○ No ○ I'm not sure

Write your other categories from last cycle below and use symbols for "More," "Less," and "I'm not sure."

(+) More   (−) Less   (?) I'm not sure

Are categories more or less present during the bleeding phase of your cycle?

_____○_____○_____○_____○_____○

What categories seem to be more or less present when you notice slippery cervical fluid?

_____○_____○_____○_____○_____○

What categories seem to be more or less present right before your next bleeding phase?

_____○_____○_____○_____○_____○

GENERAL MOOD

Are you getting what you need out of tracking?

○ Yes, this is totally working   ○ I think I'm onto something   ○ Not yet, finding more support feels like a good next step

What patterns are you curious about for your next cycle?

_____

Which categories appear unrelated to phases of your cycle?

_____

CATEGORY INSIGHTS

Write your categories from last cycle below and use symbols for keeping, refining, and dropping those descriptions.

Do any categories need a bit of refining?   What categories are you going to track next cycle?

✔ Keep   → Refine   ✗ Drop

_____   ○   _____

_____   ○   _____

_____   ○   _____

_____   ○   _____

_____   ○   _____

CYCLE PREVIEW

What are your 3 goals for this next cycle of tracking?

_____   _____   _____

What will you do differently for your next cycle?

_____

_____

What are 2 ways you can introduce comfort, safety, and/or pleasure into your cycle?

_____   _____

What are 2 ways you can make cycle tracking easier for you?

_____   _____

CYCLE

MONTH _____ DATE ___ ___ ___ ___ ___ ___ ___ ___ ___ ___ ___ ___ ___ ___ ___ ___ ___ ___

BASAL BODY TEMPERATURES

Higher Baseline BBT — _____ F/C

CYCLE DAY	1	2	3	4	5	6	7	8	9	10	11	12	13	14	15	16	17	18	19	20
9	9	9	9	9	9	9	9	9	9	9	9	9	9	9	9	9	9	9	9	9
8	8	8	8	8	8	8	8	8	8	8	8	8	8	8	8	8	8	8	8	8
7	7	7	7	7	7	7	7	7	7	7	7	7	7	7	7	7	7	7	7	7
6	6	6	6	6	6	6	6	6	6	6	6	6	6	6	6	6	6	6	6	6
5	5	5	5	5	5	5	5	5	5	5	5	5	5	5	5	5	5	5	5	5
4	4	4	4	4	4	4	4	4	4	4	4	4	4	4	4	4	4	4	4	4
3	3	3	3	3	3	3	3	3	3	3	3	3	3	3	3	3	3	3	3	3
2	2	2	2	2	2	2	2	2	2	2	2	2	2	2	2	2	2	2	2	2
1	1	1	1	1	1	1	1	1	1	1	1	1	1	1	1	1	1	1	1	1
0	0	0	0	0	0	0	0	0	0	0	0	0	0	0	0	0	0	0	0	0

Lower Baseline BBT — _____ F/C

9	9	9	9	9	9	9	9	9	9	9	9	9	9	9	9	9	9	9	9
8	8	8	8	8	8	8	8	8	8	8	8	8	8	8	8	8	8	8	8
7	7	7	7	7	7	7	7	7	7	7	7	7	7	7	7	7	7	7	7
6	6	6	6	6	6	6	6	6	6	6	6	6	6	6	6	6	6	6	6
5	5	5	5	5	5	5	5	5	5	5	5	5	5	5	5	5	5	5	5
4	4	4	4	4	4	4	4	4	4	4	4	4	4	4	4	4	4	4	4
3	3	3	3	3	3	3	3	3	3	3	3	3	3	3	3	3	3	3	3
2	2	2	2	2	2	2	2	2	2	2	2	2	2	2	2	2	2	2	2
1	1	1	1	1	1	1	1	1	1	1	1	1	1	1	1	1	1	1	1
0	0	0	0	0	0	0	0	0	0	0	0	0	0	0	0	0	0	0	0

BODY FLUIDS

CYCLE DAY	1	2	3	4	5	6	7	8	9	10	11	12	13	14	15	16	17	18	19	20
Bleeding	O	O	O	O	O	O	O	O	O	O	O	O	O	O	O	O	O	O	O	O
Spotting	O	O	O	O	O	O	O	O	O	O	O	O	O	O	O	O	O	O	O	O
Dry	O	O	O	O	O	O	O	O	O	O	O	O	O	O	O	O	O	O	O	O
Creamy	O	O	O	O	O	O	O	O	O	O	O	O	O	O	O	O	O	O	O	O
Slippery	O	O	O	O	O	O	O	O	O	O	O	O	O	O	O	O	O	O	O	O

CATEGORIES

CYCLE DAY	1	2	3	4	5	6	7	8	9	10	11	12	13	14	15	16	17	18	19	20
1 Comfort	O	O	O	O	O	O	O	O	O	O	O	O	O	O	O	O	O	O	O	O
2	O	O	O	O	O	O	O	O	O	O	O	O	O	O	O	O	O	O	O	O
3	O	O	O	O	O	O	O	O	O	O	O	O	O	O	O	O	O	O	O	O
4	O	O	O	O	O	O	O	O	O	O	O	O	O	O	O	O	O	O	O	O
5	O	O	O	O	O	O	O	O	O	O	O	O	O	O	O	O	O	O	O	O
	O	O	O	O	O	O	O	O	O	O	O	O	O	O	O	O	O	O	O	O
	O	O	O	O	O	O	O	O	O	O	O	O	O	O	O	O	O	O	O	O
6	O	O	O	O	O	O	O	O	O	O	O	O	O	O	O	O	O	O	O	O

BASAL BODY TEMPERATURES

| 21 | 22 | 23 | 24 | 25 | 26 | 27 | 28 | 29 | 30 | 31 | 32 | 33 | 34 | 35 | 36 | 37 | 38 | 39 | 40 | CYCLE DAY |

Higher Baseline BBT _____ F/C

Each column (cycle days 21–40) contains the digits 9, 8, 7, 6, 5, 4, 3, 2, 1, 0 in circles.

Lower Baseline BBT _____ F/C

Each column (cycle days 21–40) contains the digits 9, 8, 7, 6, 5, 4, 3, 2, 1, 0 in circles.

BODY FLUIDS

21	22	23	24	25	26	27	28	29	30	31	32	33	34	35	36	37	38	39	40	CYCLE DAY
O	O	O	O	O	O	O	O	O	O	O	O	O	O	O	O	O	O	O	O	Bleeding
O	O	O	O	O	O	O	O	O	O	O	O	O	O	O	O	O	O	O	O	Spotting
O	O	O	O	O	O	O	O	O	O	O	O	O	O	O	O	O	O	O	O	Dry
O	O	O	O	O	O	O	O	O	O	O	O	O	O	O	O	O	O	O	O	Creamy
O	O	O	O	O	O	O	O	O	O	O	O	O	O	O	O	O	O	O	O	Slippery

CATEGORIES

21	22	23	24	25	26	27	28	29	30	31	32	33	34	35	36	37	38	39	40	CYCLE DAY	
O	O	O	O	O	O	O	O	O	O	O	O	O	O	O	O	O	O	O	O	Comfort	1
O	O	O	O	O	O	O	O	O	O	O	O	O	O	O	O	O	O	O	O		2
O	O	O	O	O	O	O	O	O	O	O	O	O	O	O	O	O	O	O	O		3
O	O	O	O	O	O	O	O	O	O	O	O	O	O	O	O	O	O	O	O		4
O	O	O	O	O	O	O	O	O	O	O	O	O	O	O	O	O	O	O	O		
O	O	O	O	O	O	O	O	O	O	O	O	O	O	O	O	O	O	O	O		5
O	O	O	O	O	O	O	O	O	O	O	O	O	O	O	O	O	O	O	O		
O	O	O	O	O	O	O	O	O	O	O	O	O	O	O	O	O	O	O	O		
O	O	O	O	O	O	O	O	O	O	O	O	O	O	O	O	O	O	O	O		
O	O	O	O	O	O	O	O	O	O	O	O	O	O	O	O	O	O	O	O		6

CYCLE REVIEW

Analyze your last cycle and prepare for your next

BASELINE INSIGHTS

BASAL BODY TEMPERATURE

Can you identify a significant and sustained temperature increase and the day it began? ○ Yes ○ No ○ I'm not sure

_____

_____

BODY FLUID

Can you identify which day you experienced the most slippery fluid for this last cycle?   ○ Yes ○ No ○ I'm not sure

_____

_____

Could you easily differentiate bleeding and spotting for this last cycle?   ○ Yes ○ No ○ I'm not sure

_____

_____

Did you notice other body fluids during this last cycle?   ○ Yes ○ No ○ I'm not sure

_____

_____

PATTERNS

Starting with comfort, review your list of categories tracked last cycle.

Were you able to identify feelings of *comfort* during your last cycle?   ○ Yes ○ No ○ I'm not sure

Did you notice a change in how you felt on the days when comfort was present?   ○ Yes ○ No ○ I'm not sure

Write your other categories from last cycle below and use symbols for "More," "Less," and "I'm not sure."

(+) More   (−) Less   (?) I'm not sure

Are categories more or less present during the bleeding phase of your cycle?

_____○_____ _____○_____ _____○_____ _____○_____ _____○_____

What categories seem to be more or less present when you notice slippery cervical fluid?

_____○_____ _____○_____ _____○_____ _____○_____ _____○_____

What categories seem to be more or less present right before your next bleeding phase?

_____○_____ _____○_____ _____○_____ _____○_____ _____○_____

GENERAL MOOD

Are you getting what you need out of tracking?

○ Yes, this is totally working ○ I think I'm onto something ○ Not yet, finding more support feels like a good next step

What patterns are you curious about for your next cycle?

_____

Which categories appear unrelated to phases of your cycle?

_____

CATEGORY INSIGHTS

Write your categories from last cycle below and use symbols for keeping, refining, and dropping those descriptions.

Do any categories need a bit of refining?   What categories are you going to track next cycle?

(✔) Keep   (→) Refine   (✗) Drop

_____ ○ _____
_____ ○ _____
_____ ○ _____
_____ ○ _____
_____ ○ _____

CYCLE PREVIEW

What are your 3 goals for this next cycle of tracking?

_____ _____ _____

What will you do differently for your next cycle?

_____

What are 2 ways you can introduce comfort, safety, and/or pleasure into your cycle?

_____ _____

What are 2 ways you can make cycle tracking easier for you?

_____ _____

CYCLE

MONTH __________ DATE __

BASAL BODY TEMPERATURES

____F/C

Higher Baseline BBT

CYCLE DAY	1	2	3	4	5	6	7	8	9	10	11	12	13	14	15	16	17	18	19	20
	9	9	9	9	9	9	9	9	9	9	9	9	9	9	9	9	9	9	9	9
	8	8	8	8	8	8	8	8	8	8	8	8	8	8	8	8	8	8	8	8
	7	7	7	7	7	7	7	7	7	7	7	7	7	7	7	7	7	7	7	7
	6	6	6	6	6	6	6	6	6	6	6	6	6	6	6	6	6	6	6	6
	5	5	5	5	5	5	5	5	5	5	5	5	5	5	5	5	5	5	5	5
	4	4	4	4	4	4	4	4	4	4	4	4	4	4	4	4	4	4	4	4
	3	3	3	3	3	3	3	3	3	3	3	3	3	3	3	3	3	3	3	3
	2	2	2	2	2	2	2	2	2	2	2	2	2	2	2	2	2	2	2	2
	1	1	1	1	1	1	1	1	1	1	1	1	1	1	1	1	1	1	1	1
	0	0	0	0	0	0	0	0	0	0	0	0	0	0	0	0	0	0	0	0

____F/C

Lower Baseline BBT

	9	9	9	9	9	9	9	9	9	9	9	9	9	9	9	9	9	9	9	9
	8	8	8	8	8	8	8	8	8	8	8	8	8	8	8	8	8	8	8	8
	7	7	7	7	7	7	7	7	7	7	7	7	7	7	7	7	7	7	7	7
	6	6	6	6	6	6	6	6	6	6	6	6	6	6	6	6	6	6	6	6
	5	5	5	5	5	5	5	5	5	5	5	5	5	5	5	5	5	5	5	5
	4	4	4	4	4	4	4	4	4	4	4	4	4	4	4	4	4	4	4	4
	3	3	3	3	3	3	3	3	3	3	3	3	3	3	3	3	3	3	3	3
	2	2	2	2	2	2	2	2	2	2	2	2	2	2	2	2	2	2	2	2
	1	1	1	1	1	1	1	1	1	1	1	1	1	1	1	1	1	1	1	1
	0	0	0	0	0	0	0	0	0	0	0	0	0	0	0	0	0	0	0	0

BODY FLUIDS

CYCLE DAY	1	2	3	4	5	6	7	8	9	10	11	12	13	14	15	16	17	18	19	20
Bleeding	○	○	○	○	○	○	○	○	○	○	○	○	○	○	○	○	○	○	○	○
Spotting	○	○	○	○	○	○	○	○	○	○	○	○	○	○	○	○	○	○	○	○
Dry	○	○	○	○	○	○	○	○	○	○	○	○	○	○	○	○	○	○	○	○
Creamy	○	○	○	○	○	○	○	○	○	○	○	○	○	○	○	○	○	○	○	○
Slippery	○	○	○	○	○	○	○	○	○	○	○	○	○	○	○	○	○	○	○	○

CATEGORIES

CYCLE DAY	1	2	3	4	5	6	7	8	9	10	11	12	13	14	15	16	17	18	19	20
1 Comfort	○	○	○	○	○	○	○	○	○	○	○	○	○	○	○	○	○	○	○	○
2	○	○	○	○	○	○	○	○	○	○	○	○	○	○	○	○	○	○	○	○
3	○	○	○	○	○	○	○	○	○	○	○	○	○	○	○	○	○	○	○	○
4	○	○	○	○	○	○	○	○	○	○	○	○	○	○	○	○	○	○	○	○
5	○ ○ ○	○ ○ ○	○ ○ ○	○ ○ ○	○ ○ ○	○ ○ ○	○ ○ ○	○ ○ ○	○ ○ ○	○ ○ ○	○ ○ ○	○ ○ ○	○ ○ ○	○ ○ ○	○ ○ ○	○ ○ ○	○ ○ ○	○ ○ ○	○ ○ ○	○ ○ ○
6	○ ○ ○	○ ○ ○	○ ○ ○	○ ○ ○	○ ○ ○	○ ○ ○	○ ○ ○	○ ○ ○	○ ○ ○	○ ○ ○	○ ○ ○	○ ○ ○	○ ○ ○	○ ○ ○	○ ○ ○	○ ○ ○	○ ○ ○	○ ○ ○	○ ○ ○	○ ○ ○

BASIC BODY TEMPERATURES

CYCLE DAY	21	22	23	24	25	26	27	28	29	30	31	32	33	34	35	36	37	38	39	40

Higher Baseline BBT — values 9 8 7 6 5 4 3 2 1 0 repeated for each cycle day column. _____ F/C

Lower Baseline BBT — values 9 8 7 6 5 4 3 2 1 0 repeated for each cycle day column. _____ F/C

BODY FLUIDS

CYCLE DAY	21	22	23	24	25	26	27	28	29	30	31	32	33	34	35	36	37	38	39	40	
	O	O	O	O	O	O	O	O	O	O	O	O	O	O	O	O	O	O	O	O	Bleeding
	O	O	O	O	O	O	O	O	O	O	O	O	O	O	O	O	O	O	O	O	Spotting
	O	O	O	O	O	O	O	O	O	O	O	O	O	O	O	O	O	O	O	O	Dry
	O	O	O	O	O	O	O	O	O	O	O	O	O	O	O	O	O	O	O	O	Creamy
	O	O	O	O	O	O	O	O	O	O	O	O	O	O	O	O	O	O	O	O	Slippery

CATEGORIES

CYCLE DAY	21	22	23	24	25	26	27	28	29	30	31	32	33	34	35	36	37	38	39	40	
	O	O	O	O	O	O	O	O	O	O	O	O	O	O	O	O	O	O	O	O	Comfort 1
	O	O	O	O	O	O	O	O	O	O	O	O	O	O	O	O	O	O	O	O	2
	O	O	O	O	O	O	O	O	O	O	O	O	O	O	O	O	O	O	O	O	3
	O	O	O	O	O	O	O	O	O	O	O	O	O	O	O	O	O	O	O	O	4
	O	O	O	O	O	O	O	O	O	O	O	O	O	O	O	O	O	O	O	O	
	O	O	O	O	O	O	O	O	O	O	O	O	O	O	O	O	O	O	O	O	
	O	O	O	O	O	O	O	O	O	O	O	O	O	O	O	O	O	O	O	O	5
	O	O	O	O	O	O	O	O	O	O	O	O	O	O	O	O	O	O	O	O	
	O	O	O	O	O	O	O	O	O	O	O	O	O	O	O	O	O	O	O	O	
	O	O	O	O	O	O	O	O	O	O	O	O	O	O	O	O	O	O	O	O	6

CYCLE REVIEW

Analyze your last cycle and prepare for your next

BASELINE INSIGHTS

BASAL BODY TEMPERATURE

Can you identify a significant and sustained temperature increase and the day it began?　○ Yes　○ No　○ I'm not sure

_____

_____

BODY FLUID

Can you identify which day you experienced the most slippery fluid for this last cycle?　　○ Yes　○ No　○ I'm not sure

_____

_____

Could you easily differentiate bleeding and spotting for this last cycle?　　　　○ Yes　○ No　○ I'm not sure

_____

_____

Did you notice other body fluids during this last cycle?　　　　　　　○ Yes　○ No　○ I'm not sure

_____

_____

PATTERNS

Starting with comfort, review your list of categories tracked last cycle.

Were you able to identify feelings of *comfort* during your last cycle?　　　○ Yes　○ No　○ I'm not sure

Did you notice a change in how you felt on the days when comfort was present?　　○ Yes　○ No　○ I'm not sure

Write your other categories from last cycle below and use symbols for "More," "Less," and "I'm not sure."

(+) More　　(−) Less　　(?) I'm not sure

Are categories more or less present during the bleeding phase of your cycle?

____○_____○_____○_____○_____○____

What categories seem to be more or less present when you notice slippery cervical fluid?

____○_____○_____○_____○_____○____

What categories seem to be more or less present right before your next bleeding phase?

____○_____○_____○_____○_____○____

GENERAL MOOD

Are you getting what you need out of tracking?

○ Yes, this is totally working ○ I think I'm onto something ○ Not yet, finding more support feels like a good next step

What patterns are you curious about for your next cycle?

_____

Which categories appear unrelated to phases of your cycle?

_____

CATEGORY INSIGHTS

Write your categories from last cycle below and use symbols for keeping, refining, and dropping those descriptions.

Do any categories need a bit of refining?　　　　What categories are you going to track next cycle?

(✔) Keep　(→) Refine　(✗) Drop

_____　○　_____

_____　○　_____

_____　○　_____

_____　○　_____

_____　○　_____

CYCLE PREVIEW

What are your 3 goals for this next cycle of tracking?

_____　_____　_____

What will you do differently for your next cycle?

_____

_____

What are 2 ways you can introduce comfort, safety, and/or pleasure into your cycle?

_____　_____

What are 2 ways you can make cycle tracking easier for you?

_____　_____

CYCLE

MONTH _____ DATE ___

BASAL BODY TEMPERATURES

CYCLE DAY	1	2	3	4	5	6	7	8	9	10	11	12	13	14	15	16	17	18	19	20

_____ F/C — Higher Baseline BBT

Rows of bubbles numbered 9, 8, 7, 6, 5, 4, 3, 2, 1, 0 for each cycle day 1–20.

_____ F/C — Lower Baseline BBT

Rows of bubbles numbered 9, 8, 7, 6, 5, 4, 3, 2, 1, 0 for each cycle day 1–20.

BODY FLUIDS

CYCLE DAY	1	2	3	4	5	6	7	8	9	10	11	12	13	14	15	16	17	18	19	20
Bleeding	O	O	O	O	O	O	O	O	O	O	O	O	O	O	O	O	O	O	O	O
Spotting	O	O	O	O	O	O	O	O	O	O	O	O	O	O	O	O	O	O	O	O
Dry	O	O	O	O	O	O	O	O	O	O	O	O	O	O	O	O	O	O	O	O
Creamy	O	O	O	O	O	O	O	O	O	O	O	O	O	O	O	O	O	O	O	O
Slippery	O	O	O	O	O	O	O	O	O	O	O	O	O	O	O	O	O	O	O	O

CATEGORIES

CYCLE DAY	1	2	3	4	5	6	7	8	9	10	11	12	13	14	15	16	17	18	19	20
1 Comfort	O	O	O	O	O	O	O	O	O	O	O	O	O	O	O	O	O	O	O	O
2	O	O	O	O	O	O	O	O	O	O	O	O	O	O	O	O	O	O	O	O
3	O	O	O	O	O	O	O	O	O	O	O	O	O	O	O	O	O	O	O	O
4	O	O	O	O	O	O	O	O	O	O	O	O	O	O	O	O	O	O	O	O
5	O	O	O	O	O	O	O	O	O	O	O	O	O	O	O	O	O	O	O	O
	O	O	O	O	O	O	O	O	O	O	O	O	O	O	O	O	O	O	O	O
6	O	O	O	O	O	O	O	O	O	O	O	O	O	O	O	O	O	O	O	O
	O	O	O	O	O	O	O	O	O	O	O	O	O	O	O	O	O	O	O	O

______ DATE ______ MONTH

BASAL BODY TEMPERATURES

21	22	23	24	25	26	27	28	29	30	31	32	33	34	35	36	37	38	39	40	CYCLE DAY
9	9	9	9	9	9	9	9	9	9	9	9	9	9	9	9	9	9	9	9	Higher Baseline BBT
8	8	8	8	8	8	8	8	8	8	8	8	8	8	8	8	8	8	8	8	
7	7	7	7	7	7	7	7	7	7	7	7	7	7	7	7	7	7	7	7	
6	6	6	6	6	6	6	6	6	6	6	6	6	6	6	6	6	6	6	6	
5	5	5	5	5	5	5	5	5	5	5	5	5	5	5	5	5	5	5	5	______ F/C
4	4	4	4	4	4	4	4	4	4	4	4	4	4	4	4	4	4	4	4	
3	3	3	3	3	3	3	3	3	3	3	3	3	3	3	3	3	3	3	3	
2	2	2	2	2	2	2	2	2	2	2	2	2	2	2	2	2	2	2	2	
1	1	1	1	1	1	1	1	1	1	1	1	1	1	1	1	1	1	1	1	
0	0	0	0	0	0	0	0	0	0	0	0	0	0	0	0	0	0	0	0	
9	9	9	9	9	9	9	9	9	9	9	9	9	9	9	9	9	9	9	9	Lower Baseline BBT
8	8	8	8	8	8	8	8	8	8	8	8	8	8	8	8	8	8	8	8	
7	7	7	7	7	7	7	7	7	7	7	7	7	7	7	7	7	7	7	7	
6	6	6	6	6	6	6	6	6	6	6	6	6	6	6	6	6	6	6	6	
5	5	5	5	5	5	5	5	5	5	5	5	5	5	5	5	5	5	5	5	______ F/C
4	4	4	4	4	4	4	4	4	4	4	4	4	4	4	4	4	4	4	4	
3	3	3	3	3	3	3	3	3	3	3	3	3	3	3	3	3	3	3	3	
2	2	2	2	2	2	2	2	2	2	2	2	2	2	2	2	2	2	2	2	
1	1	1	1	1	1	1	1	1	1	1	1	1	1	1	1	1	1	1	1	
0	0	0	0	0	0	0	0	0	0	0	0	0	0	0	0	0	0	0	0	

BODY FLUIDS

21	22	23	24	25	26	27	28	29	30	31	32	33	34	35	36	37	38	39	40	CYCLE DAY
O	O	O	O	O	O	O	O	O	O	O	O	O	O	O	O	O	O	O	O	Bleeding
O	O	O	O	O	O	O	O	O	O	O	O	O	O	O	O	O	O	O	O	Spotting
O	O	O	O	O	O	O	O	O	O	O	O	O	O	O	O	O	O	O	O	Dry
O	O	O	O	O	O	O	O	O	O	O	O	O	O	O	O	O	O	O	O	Creamy
O	O	O	O	O	O	O	O	O	O	O	O	O	O	O	O	O	O	O	O	Slippery

CATEGORIES

21	22	23	24	25	26	27	28	29	30	31	32	33	34	35	36	37	38	39	40	CYCLE DAY	
O	O	O	O	O	O	O	O	O	O	O	O	O	O	O	O	O	O	O	O	Comfort	1
O	O	O	O	O	O	O	O	O	O	O	O	O	O	O	O	O	O	O	O		2
O	O	O	O	O	O	O	O	O	O	O	O	O	O	O	O	O	O	O	O		3
O	O	O	O	O	O	O	O	O	O	O	O	O	O	O	O	O	O	O	O		4
O	O	O	O	O	O	O	O	O	O	O	O	O	O	O	O	O	O	O	O		
O	O	O	O	O	O	O	O	O	O	O	O	O	O	O	O	O	O	O	O		
O	O	O	O	O	O	O	O	O	O	O	O	O	O	O	O	O	O	O	O		5
O	O	O	O	O	O	O	O	O	O	O	O	O	O	O	O	O	O	O	O		
O	O	O	O	O	O	O	O	O	O	O	O	O	O	O	O	O	O	O	O		
O	O	O	O	O	O	O	O	O	O	O	O	O	O	O	O	O	O	O	O		6

CYCLE REVIEW

Analyze your last cycle and prepare for your next

BASELINE INSIGHTS

BASAL BODY TEMPERATURE

Can you identify a significant and sustained temperature increase and the day it began?　○ Yes　○ No　○ I'm not sure

_____

_____

BODY FLUID

Can you identify which day you experienced the most slippery fluid for this last cycle?　　○ Yes　○ No　○ I'm not sure

_____

_____

Could you easily differentiate bleeding and spotting for this last cycle?　　○ Yes　○ No　○ I'm not sure

_____

_____

Did you notice other body fluids during this last cycle?　　○ Yes　○ No　○ I'm not sure

_____

_____

PATTERNS

*Starting with **comfort**, review your list of categories tracked last cycle.*

Were you able to identify feelings of *comfort* during your last cycle?　　○ Yes　○ No　○ I'm not sure

Did you notice a change in how you felt on the days when comfort was present?　　○ Yes　○ No　○ I'm not sure

Write your other categories from last cycle below and use symbols for "More," "Less," and "I'm not sure."

(+) More　(−) Less　(?) I'm not sure

Are categories more or less present during the bleeding phase of your cycle?

____○____○____○____○____○

What categories seem to be more or less present when you notice slippery cervical fluid?

____○____○____○____○____○

What categories seem to be more or less present right before your next bleeding phase?

____○____○____○____○____○

GENERAL MOOD

Are you getting what you need out of tracking?

○ Yes, this is totally working   ○ I think I'm onto something   ○ Not yet, finding more support feels like a good next step

What patterns are you curious about for your next cycle?

_____

Which categories appear unrelated to phases of your cycle?

_____

CATEGORY INSIGHTS

Write your categories from last cycle below and use symbols for keeping, refining, and dropping those descriptions.

Do any categories need a bit of refining?   What categories are you going to track next cycle?

(✔) Keep   (→) Refine   (✗) Drop

_____   ○   _____

_____   ○   _____

_____   ○   _____

_____   ○   _____

_____   ○   _____

CYCLE PREVIEW

What are your 3 goals for this next cycle of tracking?

_____   _____   _____

What will you do differently for your next cycle?

_____

_____

What are 2 ways you can introduce comfort, safety, and/or pleasure into your cycle?

_____   _____

What are 2 ways you can make cycle tracking easier for you?

_____   _____

CYCLE

BASAL BODY TEMPERATURES

CYCLE DAY 1 2 3 4 5 6 7 8 9 10 11 12 13 14 15 16 17 18 19 20

_____ F/C — Higher Baseline BBT

Values 9 8 7 6 5 4 3 2 1 0 for each cycle day

_____ F/C — Lower Baseline BBT

Values 9 8 7 6 5 4 3 2 1 0 for each cycle day

BODY FLUIDS

CYCLE DAY 1 2 3 4 5 6 7 8 9 10 11 12 13 14 15 16 17 18 19 20

Bleeding	○	○	○	○	○	○	○	○	○	○	○	○	○	○	○	○	○	○	○	○
Spotting	○	○	○	○	○	○	○	○	○	○	○	○	○	○	○	○	○	○	○	○
Dry	○	○	○	○	○	○	○	○	○	○	○	○	○	○	○	○	○	○	○	○
Creamy	○	○	○	○	○	○	○	○	○	○	○	○	○	○	○	○	○	○	○	○
Slippery	○	○	○	○	○	○	○	○	○	○	○	○	○	○	○	○	○	○	○	○

CATEGORIES

CYCLE DAY 1 2 3 4 5 6 7 8 9 10 11 12 13 14 15 16 17 18 19 20

1 Comfort	○	○	○	○	○	○	○	○	○	○	○	○	○	○	○	○	○	○	○	○
2	○	○	○	○	○	○	○	○	○	○	○	○	○	○	○	○	○	○	○	○
3	○	○	○	○	○	○	○	○	○	○	○	○	○	○	○	○	○	○	○	○
4	○	○	○	○	○	○	○	○	○	○	○	○	○	○	○	○	○	○	○	○
5	○	○	○	○	○	○	○	○	○	○	○	○	○	○	○	○	○	○	○	○
5	○	○	○	○	○	○	○	○	○	○	○	○	○	○	○	○	○	○	○	○
6	○	○	○	○	○	○	○	○	○	○	○	○	○	○	○	○	○	○	○	○
6	○	○	○	○	○	○	○	○	○	○	○	○	○	○	○	○	○	○	○	○

BASAL BODY TEMPERATURES

CYCLE DAY	21	22	23	24	25	26	27	28	29	30	31	32	33	34	35	36	37	38	39	40

Higher Baseline BBT _____ F/C

9 8 7 6 5 4 3 2 1 0 (columns 21–40)

Lower Baseline BBT _____ F/C

9 8 7 6 5 4 3 2 1 0 (columns 21–40)

BODY FLUIDS

CYCLE DAY	21	22	23	24	25	26	27	28	29	30	31	32	33	34	35	36	37	38	39	40	
O	O	O	O	O	O	O	O	O	O	O	O	O	O	O	O	O	O	O	O	Bleeding
O	O	O	O	O	O	O	O	O	O	O	O	O	O	O	O	O	O	O	O	Spotting
O	O	O	O	O	O	O	O	O	O	O	O	O	O	O	O	O	O	O	O	Dry
O	O	O	O	O	O	O	O	O	O	O	O	O	O	O	O	O	O	O	O	Creamy
O	O	O	O	O	O	O	O	O	O	O	O	O	O	O	O	O	O	O	O	Slippery

CATEGORIES

CYCLE DAY	21	22	23	24	25	26	27	28	29	30	31	32	33	34	35	36	37	38	39	40		
O	O	O	O	O	O	O	O	O	O	O	O	O	O	O	O	O	O	O	O	Comfort	1
O	O	O	O	O	O	O	O	O	O	O	O	O	O	O	O	O	O	O	O		2
O	O	O	O	O	O	O	O	O	O	O	O	O	O	O	O	O	O	O	O		3
O	O	O	O	O	O	O	O	O	O	O	O	O	O	O	O	O	O	O	O		4
O	O	O	O	O	O	O	O	O	O	O	O	O	O	O	O	O	O	O	O		
O	O	O	O	O	O	O	O	O	O	O	O	O	O	O	O	O	O	O	O		
O	O	O	O	O	O	O	O	O	O	O	O	O	O	O	O	O	O	O	O		5
O	O	O	O	O	O	O	O	O	O	O	O	O	O	O	O	O	O	O	O		
O	O	O	O	O	O	O	O	O	O	O	O	O	O	O	O	O	O	O	O		
O	O	O	O	O	O	O	O	O	O	O	O	O	O	O	O	O	O	O	O		6

CYCLE REVIEW

Analyze your last cycle and prepare for your next

BASELINE INSIGHTS

BASAL BODY TEMPERATURE

Can you identify a significant and sustained temperature increase and the day it began?   ○ Yes ○ No ○ I'm not sure

_____

_____

BODY FLUID

Can you identify which day you experienced the most slippery fluid for this last cycle?   ○ Yes ○ No ○ I'm not sure

_____

_____

Could you easily differentiate bleeding and spotting for this last cycle?   ○ Yes ○ No ○ I'm not sure

_____

_____

Did you notice other body fluids during this last cycle?   ○ Yes ○ No ○ I'm not sure

_____

_____

PATTERNS

*Starting with **comfort**, review your list of categories tracked last cycle.*

Were you able to identify feelings of *comfort* during your last cycle?   ○ Yes ○ No ○ I'm not sure

Did you notice a change in how you felt on the days when comfort was present?   ○ Yes ○ No ○ I'm not sure

Write your other categories from last cycle below and use symbols for "More," "Less," and "I'm not sure."

(+) More   (−) Less   (?) I'm not sure

Are categories more or less present during the bleeding phase of your cycle?

___ ○ ___ ○ ___ ○ ___ ○ ___ ○

What categories seem to be more or less present when you notice slippery cervical fluid?

___ ○ ___ ○ ___ ○ ___ ○ ___ ○

What categories seem to be more or less present right before your next bleeding phase?

___ ○ ___ ○ ___ ○ ___ ○ ___ ○

GENERAL MOOD

Are you getting what you need out of tracking?

○ Yes, this is totally working   ○ I think I'm onto something   ○ Not yet, finding more support feels like a good next step

What patterns are you curious about for your next cycle?

_____

Which categories appear unrelated to phases of your cycle?

_____

CATEGORY INSIGHTS

Write your categories from last cycle below and use symbols for keeping, refining, and dropping those descriptions.

Do any categories need a bit of refining?   What categories are you going to track next cycle?

(✔) Keep   (→) Refine   (✗) Drop

_____   ○   _____
_____   ○   _____
_____   ○   _____
_____   ○   _____
_____   ○   _____

CYCLE PREVIEW

What are your 3 goals for this next cycle of tracking?

_____   _____   _____

What will you do differently for your next cycle?

_____

_____

What are 2 ways you can introduce comfort, safety, and/or pleasure into your cycle?

_____   _____

What are 2 ways you can make cycle tracking easier for you?

_____   _____

CYCLE

MONTH _____ DATE ___ ___ ___ ___ ___ ___ ___ ___ ___ ___ ___

BASAL BODY TEMPERATURES

Higher Baseline BBT — ___ F/C

CYCLE DAY	1	2	3	4	5	6	7	8	9	10	11	12	13	14	15	16	17	18	19	20
	9	9	9	9	9	9	9	9	9	9	9	9	9	9	9	9	9	9	9	9
	8	8	8	8	8	8	8	8	8	8	8	8	8	8	8	8	8	8	8	8
	7	7	7	7	7	7	7	7	7	7	7	7	7	7	7	7	7	7	7	7
	6	6	6	6	6	6	6	6	6	6	6	6	6	6	6	6	6	6	6	6
	5	5	5	5	5	5	5	5	5	5	5	5	5	5	5	5	5	5	5	5
	4	4	4	4	4	4	4	4	4	4	4	4	4	4	4	4	4	4	4	4
	3	3	3	3	3	3	3	3	3	3	3	3	3	3	3	3	3	3	3	3
	2	2	2	2	2	2	2	2	2	2	2	2	2	2	2	2	2	2	2	2
	1	1	1	1	1	1	1	1	1	1	1	1	1	1	1	1	1	1	1	1
	0	0	0	0	0	0	0	0	0	0	0	0	0	0	0	0	0	0	0	0

Lower Baseline BBT — ___ F/C

CYCLE DAY	1	2	3	4	5	6	7	8	9	10	11	12	13	14	15	16	17	18	19	20
	9	9	9	9	9	9	9	9	9	9	9	9	9	9	9	9	9	9	9	9
	8	8	8	8	8	8	8	8	8	8	8	8	8	8	8	8	8	8	8	8
	7	7	7	7	7	7	7	7	7	7	7	7	7	7	7	7	7	7	7	7
	6	6	6	6	6	6	6	6	6	6	6	6	6	6	6	6	6	6	6	6
	5	5	5	5	5	5	5	5	5	5	5	5	5	5	5	5	5	5	5	5
	4	4	4	4	4	4	4	4	4	4	4	4	4	4	4	4	4	4	4	4
	3	3	3	3	3	3	3	3	3	3	3	3	3	3	3	3	3	3	3	3
	2	2	2	2	2	2	2	2	2	2	2	2	2	2	2	2	2	2	2	2
	1	1	1	1	1	1	1	1	1	1	1	1	1	1	1	1	1	1	1	1
	0	0	0	0	0	0	0	0	0	0	0	0	0	0	0	0	0	0	0	0

BODY FLUIDS

CYCLE DAY	1	2	3	4	5	6	7	8	9	10	11	12	13	14	15	16	17	18	19	20
Bleeding	O	O	O	O	O	O	O	O	O	O	O	O	O	O	O	O	O	O	O	O
Spotting	O	O	O	O	O	O	O	O	O	O	O	O	O	O	O	O	O	O	O	O
Dry	O	O	O	O	O	O	O	O	O	O	O	O	O	O	O	O	O	O	O	O
Creamy	O	O	O	O	O	O	O	O	O	O	O	O	O	O	O	O	O	O	O	O
Slippery	O	O	O	O	O	O	O	O	O	O	O	O	O	O	O	O	O	O	O	O

CATEGORIES

CYCLE DAY		1	2	3	4	5	6	7	8	9	10	11	12	13	14	15	16	17	18	19	20
1	Comfort	O	O	O	O	O	O	O	O	O	O	O	O	O	O	O	O	O	O	O	O
2		O	O	O	O	O	O	O	O	O	O	O	O	O	O	O	O	O	O	O	O
3		O	O	O	O	O	O	O	O	O	O	O	O	O	O	O	O	O	O	O	O
4		O	O	O	O	O	O	O	O	O	O	O	O	O	O	O	O	O	O	O	O
5		O	O	O	O	O	O	O	O	O	O	O	O	O	O	O	O	O	O	O	O
		O	O	O	O	O	O	O	O	O	O	O	O	O	O	O	O	O	O	O	O
		O	O	O	O	O	O	O	O	O	O	O	O	O	O	O	O	O	O	O	O
6		O	O	O	O	O	O	O	O	O	O	O	O	O	O	O	O	O	O	O	O
		O	O	O	O	O	O	O	O	O	O	O	O	O	O	O	O	O	O	O	O
		O	O	O	O	O	O	O	O	O	O	O	O	O	O	O	O	O	O	O	O

BASAL BODY TEMPERATURES

| CYCLE DAY | 21 | 22 | 23 | 24 | 25 | 26 | 27 | 28 | 29 | 30 | 31 | 32 | 33 | 34 | 35 | 36 | 37 | 38 | 39 | 40 |

Higher Baseline BBT _____ F/C

Rows (each column contains circled digits): 9 8 7 6 5 4 3 2 1 0

Lower Baseline BBT _____ F/C

Rows (each column contains circled digits): 9 8 7 6 5 4 3 2 1 0

BODY FLUIDS

CYCLE DAY	21	22	23	24	25	26	27	28	29	30	31	32	33	34	35	36	37	38	39	40	
	○	○	○	○	○	○	○	○	○	○	○	○	○	○	○	○	○	○	○	○	Bleeding
	○	○	○	○	○	○	○	○	○	○	○	○	○	○	○	○	○	○	○	○	Spotting
	○	○	○	○	○	○	○	○	○	○	○	○	○	○	○	○	○	○	○	○	Dry
	○	○	○	○	○	○	○	○	○	○	○	○	○	○	○	○	○	○	○	○	Creamy
	○	○	○	○	○	○	○	○	○	○	○	○	○	○	○	○	○	○	○	○	Slippery

CATEGORIES

CYCLE DAY	21	22	23	24	25	26	27	28	29	30	31	32	33	34	35	36	37	38	39	40		
	○	○	○	○	○	○	○	○	○	○	○	○	○	○	○	○	○	○	○	○	Comfort	1
	○	○	○	○	○	○	○	○	○	○	○	○	○	○	○	○	○	○	○	○		2
	○	○	○	○	○	○	○	○	○	○	○	○	○	○	○	○	○	○	○	○		3
	○	○	○	○	○	○	○	○	○	○	○	○	○	○	○	○	○	○	○	○		4
	○	○	○	○	○	○	○	○	○	○	○	○	○	○	○	○	○	○	○	○		
	○	○	○	○	○	○	○	○	○	○	○	○	○	○	○	○	○	○	○	○		
	○	○	○	○	○	○	○	○	○	○	○	○	○	○	○	○	○	○	○	○		5
	○	○	○	○	○	○	○	○	○	○	○	○	○	○	○	○	○	○	○	○		
	○	○	○	○	○	○	○	○	○	○	○	○	○	○	○	○	○	○	○	○		
	○	○	○	○	○	○	○	○	○	○	○	○	○	○	○	○	○	○	○	○		6

CYCLE REVIEW

Analyze your last cycle and prepare for your next

BASELINE INSIGHTS

BASAL BODY TEMPERATURE

Can you identify a significant and sustained temperature increase and the day it began? ◯ Yes ◯ No ◯ I'm not sure

_____

_____

BODY FLUID

Can you identify which day you experienced the most slippery fluid for this last cycle? ◯ Yes ◯ No ◯ I'm not sure

_____

_____

Could you easily differentiate bleeding and spotting for this last cycle? ◯ Yes ◯ No ◯ I'm not sure

_____

_____

Did you notice other body fluids during this last cycle? ◯ Yes ◯ No ◯ I'm not sure

_____

_____

PATTERNS

Starting with comfort, review your list of categories tracked last cycle.

Were you able to identify feelings of *comfort* during your last cycle? ◯ Yes ◯ No ◯ I'm not sure

Did you notice a change in how you felt on the days when comfort was present? ◯ Yes ◯ No ◯ I'm not sure

Write your other categories from last cycle below and use symbols for "More," "Less," and "I'm not sure."

(+) More   (−) Less   (?) I'm not sure

Are categories more or less present during the bleeding phase of your cycle?

____◯____◯____◯____◯____◯

What categories seem to be more or less present when you notice slippery cervical fluid?

____◯____◯____◯____◯____◯

What categories seem to be more or less present right before your next bleeding phase?

____◯____◯____◯____◯____◯

GENERAL MOOD

Are you getting what you need out of tracking?

○ Yes, this is totally working ○ I think I'm onto something ○ Not yet, finding more support feels like a good next step

What patterns are you curious about for your next cycle?

_____

Which categories appear unrelated to phases of your cycle?

_____

CATEGORY INSIGHTS

Write your categories from last cycle below and use symbols for keeping, refining, and dropping those descriptions.

Do any categories need a bit of refining?   What categories are you going to track next cycle?

✔ Keep   → Refine   ✗ Drop

_____ ○ _____

_____ ○ _____

_____ ○ _____

_____ ○ _____

_____ ○ _____

CYCLE PREVIEW

What are your 3 goals for this next cycle of tracking?

_____ _____ _____

What will you do differently for your next cycle?

_____

_____

What are 2 ways you can introduce comfort, safety, and/or pleasure into your cycle?

_____ _____

What are 2 ways you can make cycle tracking easier for you?

_____ _____

CYCLE

MONTH _____ DATE _____ ___ ___ ___ ___ ___ ___ ___ ___ ___ ___ ___ ___

BASAL BODY TEMPERATURES

CYCLE DAY	1	2	3	4	5	6	7	8	9	10	11	12	13	14	15	16	17	18	19	20

_____ F/C — Higher Baseline BBT

Rows (each column day): 9 8 7 6 5 4 3 2 1 0

_____ F/C — Lower Baseline BBT

Rows (each column day): 9 8 7 6 5 4 3 2 1 0

BODY FLUIDS

CYCLE DAY	1	2	3	4	5	6	7	8	9	10	11	12	13	14	15	16	17	18	19	20
Bleeding	O	O	O	O	O	O	O	O	O	O	O	O	O	O	O	O	O	O	O	O
Spotting	O	O	O	O	O	O	O	O	O	O	O	O	O	O	O	O	O	O	O	O
Dry	O	O	O	O	O	O	O	O	O	O	O	O	O	O	O	O	O	O	O	O
Creamy	O	O	O	O	O	O	O	O	O	O	O	O	O	O	O	O	O	O	O	O
Slippery	O	O	O	O	O	O	O	O	O	O	O	O	O	O	O	O	O	O	O	O

CATEGORIES

CYCLE DAY	1	2	3	4	5	6	7	8	9	10	11	12	13	14	15	16	17	18	19	20
1 Comfort	O	O	O	O	O	O	O	O	O	O	O	O	O	O	O	O	O	O	O	O
2	O	O	O	O	O	O	O	O	O	O	O	O	O	O	O	O	O	O	O	O
3	O	O	O	O	O	O	O	O	O	O	O	O	O	O	O	O	O	O	O	O
4	O	O	O	O	O	O	O	O	O	O	O	O	O	O	O	O	O	O	O	O
5	O	O	O	O	O	O	O	O	O	O	O	O	O	O	O	O	O	O	O	O
	O	O	O	O	O	O	O	O	O	O	O	O	O	O	O	O	O	O	O	O
6	O	O	O	O	O	O	O	O	O	O	O	O	O	O	O	O	O	O	O	O

___ DATE __________ MONTH

BASAL BODY TEMPERATURES

21	22	23	24	25	26	27	28	29	30	31	32	33	34	35	36	37	38	39	40	CYCLE DAY
9	9	9	9	9	9	9	9	9	9	9	9	9	9	9	9	9	9	9	9	Higher Baseline BBT ____ F/C
8	8	8	8	8	8	8	8	8	8	8	8	8	8	8	8	8	8	8	8	
7	7	7	7	7	7	7	7	7	7	7	7	7	7	7	7	7	7	7	7	
6	6	6	6	6	6	6	6	6	6	6	6	6	6	6	6	6	6	6	6	
5	5	5	5	5	5	5	5	5	5	5	5	5	5	5	5	5	5	5	5	
4	4	4	4	4	4	4	4	4	4	4	4	4	4	4	4	4	4	4	4	
3	3	3	3	3	3	3	3	3	3	3	3	3	3	3	3	3	3	3	3	
2	2	2	2	2	2	2	2	2	2	2	2	2	2	2	2	2	2	2	2	
1	1	1	1	1	1	1	1	1	1	1	1	1	1	1	1	1	1	1	1	
0	0	0	0	0	0	0	0	0	0	0	0	0	0	0	0	0	0	0	0	
9	9	9	9	9	9	9	9	9	9	9	9	9	9	9	9	9	9	9	9	Lower Baseline BBT ____ F/C
8	8	8	8	8	8	8	8	8	8	8	8	8	8	8	8	8	8	8	8	
7	7	7	7	7	7	7	7	7	7	7	7	7	7	7	7	7	7	7	7	
6	6	6	6	6	6	6	6	6	6	6	6	6	6	6	6	6	6	6	6	
5	5	5	5	5	5	5	5	5	5	5	5	5	5	5	5	5	5	5	5	
4	4	4	4	4	4	4	4	4	4	4	4	4	4	4	4	4	4	4	4	
3	3	3	3	3	3	3	3	3	3	3	3	3	3	3	3	3	3	3	3	
2	2	2	2	2	2	2	2	2	2	2	2	2	2	2	2	2	2	2	2	
1	1	1	1	1	1	1	1	1	1	1	1	1	1	1	1	1	1	1	1	
0	0	0	0	0	0	0	0	0	0	0	0	0	0	0	0	0	0	0	0	

BODY FLUIDS

21	22	23	24	25	26	27	28	29	30	31	32	33	34	35	36	37	38	39	40	CYCLE DAY
																				Bleeding
																				Spotting
																				Dry
																				Creamy
																				Slippery

CATEGORIES

21	22	23	24	25	26	27	28	29	30	31	32	33	34	35	36	37	38	39	40	CYCLE DAY
																				Comfort 1
																				2
																				3
																				4
																				5
																				6

CYCLE REVIEW

Analyze your last cycle and prepare for your next

BASELINE INSIGHTS

BASAL BODY TEMPERATURE

Can you identify a significant and sustained temperature increase and the day it began?   ○ Yes ○ No ○ I'm not sure

_____

_____

BODY FLUID

Can you identify which day you experienced the most slippery fluid for this last cycle?   ○ Yes ○ No ○ I'm not sure

_____

_____

Could you easily differentiate bleeding and spotting for this last cycle?   ○ Yes ○ No ○ I'm not sure

_____

_____

Did you notice other body fluids during this last cycle?   ○ Yes ○ No ○ I'm not sure

_____

_____

PATTERNS

Starting with comfort, *review your list of categories tracked last cycle.*

Were you able to identify feelings of *comfort* during your last cycle?   ○ Yes ○ No ○ I'm not sure

Did you notice a change in how you felt on the days when comfort was present?   ○ Yes ○ No ○ I'm not sure

Write your other categories from last cycle below and use symbols for "More," "Less," and "I'm not sure."

(+) More   (−) Less   (?) I'm not sure

Are categories more or less present during the bleeding phase of your cycle?

_____○_____○_____○_____○_____○

What categories seem to be more or less present when you notice slippery cervical fluid?

_____○_____○_____○_____○_____○

What categories seem to be more or less present right before your next bleeding phase?

_____○_____○_____○_____○_____○

GENERAL MOOD

Are you getting what you need out of tracking?

○ Yes, this is totally working   ○ I think I'm onto something   ○ Not yet, finding more support feels like a good next step

What patterns are you curious about for your next cycle?

_____

Which categories appear unrelated to phases of your cycle?

_____

CATEGORY INSIGHTS

Write your categories from last cycle below and use symbols for keeping, refining, and dropping those descriptions.

Do any categories need a bit of refining?   What categories are you going to track next cycle?

✔ Keep   → Refine   ✗ Drop

_____   ○   _____

_____   ○   _____

_____   ○   _____

_____   ○   _____

_____   ○   _____

CYCLE PREVIEW

What are your 3 goals for this next cycle of tracking?

_____   _____   _____

What will you do differently for your next cycle?

_____

_____

What are 2 ways you can introduce comfort, safety, and/or pleasure into your cycle?

_____   _____

What are 2 ways you can make cycle tracking easier for you?

_____   _____

CYCLE

MONTH _____ DATE ___ __ __ __ __ __ __ __ __ __ __ __ __ __ __ __ __ __ __ __

BASAL BODY TEMPERATURES

Higher Baseline BBT — _____ F/C

CYCLE DAY	1	2	3	4	5	6	7	8	9	10	11	12	13	14	15	16	17	18	19	20

Grid rows: 9, 8, 7, 6, 5, 4, 3, 2, 1, 0

Lower Baseline BBT — _____ F/C

Grid rows: 9, 8, 7, 6, 5, 4, 3, 2, 1, 0

BODY FLUIDS

CYCLE DAY	1	2	3	4	5	6	7	8	9	10	11	12	13	14	15	16	17	18	19	20
Bleeding	O	O	O	O	O	O	O	O	O	O	O	O	O	O	O	O	O	O	O	O
Spotting	O	O	O	O	O	O	O	O	O	O	O	O	O	O	O	O	O	O	O	O
Dry	O	O	O	O	O	O	O	O	O	O	O	O	O	O	O	O	O	O	O	O
Creamy	O	O	O	O	O	O	O	O	O	O	O	O	O	O	O	O	O	O	O	O
Slippery	O	O	O	O	O	O	O	O	O	O	O	O	O	O	O	O	O	O	O	O

CATEGORIES

CYCLE DAY	1	2	3	4	5	6	7	8	9	10	11	12	13	14	15	16	17	18	19	20
1 Comfort	O	O	O	O	O	O	O	O	O	O	O	O	O	O	O	O	O	O	O	O
2	O	O	O	O	O	O	O	O	O	O	O	O	O	O	O	O	O	O	O	O
3	O	O	O	O	O	O	O	O	O	O	O	O	O	O	O	O	O	O	O	O
4	O	O	O	O	O	O	O	O	O	O	O	O	O	O	O	O	O	O	O	O
5	O	O	O	O	O	O	O	O	O	O	O	O	O	O	O	O	O	O	O	O
5	O	O	O	O	O	O	O	O	O	O	O	O	O	O	O	O	O	O	O	O
5	O	O	O	O	O	O	O	O	O	O	O	O	O	O	O	O	O	O	O	O
6	O	O	O	O	O	O	O	O	O	O	O	O	O	O	O	O	O	O	O	O
6	O	O	O	O	O	O	O	O	O	O	O	O	O	O	O	O	O	O	O	O
6	O	O	O	O	O	O	O	O	O	O	O	O	O	O	O	O	O	O	O	O

BASAL BODY TEMPERATURES

21	22	23	24	25	26	27	28	29	30	31	32	33	34	35	36	37	38	39	40	CYCLE DAY

Higher Baseline BBT _____ F/C

(grid of values 9,8,7,6,5,4,3,2,1,0 for each cycle day)

Lower Baseline BBT _____ F/C

(grid of values 9,8,7,6,5,4,3,2,1,0 for each cycle day)

BODY FLUIDS

21	22	23	24	25	26	27	28	29	30	31	32	33	34	35	36	37	38	39	40	CYCLE DAY
O	O	O	O	O	O	O	O	O	O	O	O	O	O	O	O	O	O	O	O	Bleeding
O	O	O	O	O	O	O	O	O	O	O	O	O	O	O	O	O	O	O	O	Spotting
O	O	O	O	O	O	O	O	O	O	O	O	O	O	O	O	O	O	O	O	Dry
O	O	O	O	O	O	O	O	O	O	O	O	O	O	O	O	O	O	O	O	Creamy
O	O	O	O	O	O	O	O	O	O	O	O	O	O	O	O	O	O	O	O	Slippery

CATEGORIES

21	22	23	24	25	26	27	28	29	30	31	32	33	34	35	36	37	38	39	40	CYCLE DAY	
O	O	O	O	O	O	O	O	O	O	O	O	O	O	O	O	O	O	O	O	Comfort	1
O	O	O	O	O	O	O	O	O	O	O	O	O	O	O	O	O	O	O	O		2
O	O	O	O	O	O	O	O	O	O	O	O	O	O	O	O	O	O	O	O		3
O	O	O	O	O	O	O	O	O	O	O	O	O	O	O	O	O	O	O	O		4
O	O	O	O	O	O	O	O	O	O	O	O	O	O	O	O	O	O	O	O		
O	O	O	O	O	O	O	O	O	O	O	O	O	O	O	O	O	O	O	O		
O	O	O	O	O	O	O	O	O	O	O	O	O	O	O	O	O	O	O	O		5
O	O	O	O	O	O	O	O	O	O	O	O	O	O	O	O	O	O	O	O		
O	O	O	O	O	O	O	O	O	O	O	O	O	O	O	O	O	O	O	O		
O	O	O	O	O	O	O	O	O	O	O	O	O	O	O	O	O	O	O	O		6

CYCLE REVIEW

Analyze your last cycle and prepare for your next

BASELINE INSIGHTS

BASAL BODY TEMPERATURE

Can you identify a significant and sustained temperature increase and the day it began? ○ Yes ○ No ○ I'm not sure

_____

_____

BODY FLUID

Can you identify which day you experienced the most slippery fluid for this last cycle? ○ Yes ○ No ○ I'm not sure

_____

_____

Could you easily differentiate bleeding and spotting for this last cycle? ○ Yes ○ No ○ I'm not sure

_____

_____

Did you notice other body fluids during this last cycle? ○ Yes ○ No ○ I'm not sure

_____

_____

PATTERNS

Starting with comfort, *review your list of categories tracked last cycle.*

Were you able to identify feelings of *comfort* during your last cycle? ○ Yes ○ No ○ I'm not sure

Did you notice a change in how you felt on the days when comfort was present? ○ Yes ○ No ○ I'm not sure

Write your other categories from last cycle below and use symbols for "More," "Less," and "I'm not sure."

(+) More (−) Less (?) I'm not sure

Are categories more or less present during the bleeding phase of your cycle?

___○___ ___○___ ___○___ ___○___ ___○

What categories seem to be more or less present when you notice slippery cervical fluid?

___○___ ___○___ ___○___ ___○___ ___○

What categories seem to be more or less present right before your next bleeding phase?

___○___ ___○___ ___○___ ___○___ ___○

GENERAL MOOD

Are you getting what you need out of tracking?

○ Yes, this is totally working ○ I think I'm onto something ○ Not yet, finding more support feels like a good next step

What patterns are you curious about for your next cycle?

_____

Which categories appear unrelated to phases of your cycle?

_____

CATEGORY INSIGHTS

Write your categories from last cycle below and use symbols for keeping, refining, and dropping those descriptions.

Do any categories need a bit of refining?   What categories are you going to track next cycle?

(✔) Keep (→) Refine (✗) Drop

_____ ○ _____

_____ ○ _____

_____ ○ _____

_____ ○ _____

_____ ○

CYCLE PREVIEW

What are your 3 goals for this next cycle of tracking?

_____ _____ _____

What will you do differently for your next cycle?

_____

_____

What are 2 ways you can introduce comfort, safety, and/or pleasure into your cycle?

_____ _____

What are 2 ways you can make cycle tracking easier for you?

_____ _____

CYCLE

MONTH _____ DATE ___

BASAL BODY TEMPERATURES

CYCLE DAY	1	2	3	4	5	6	7	8	9	10	11	12	13	14	15	16	17	18	19	20

_____F/C — Higher Baseline BBT

Rows (each day column contains bubbles): 9 8 7 6 5 4 3 2 1 0

_____F/C — Lower Baseline BBT

Rows (each day column contains bubbles): 9 8 7 6 5 4 3 2 1 0

BODY FLUIDS

CYCLE DAY	1	2	3	4	5	6	7	8	9	10	11	12	13	14	15	16	17	18	19	20
Bleeding	O	O	O	O	O	O	O	O	O	O	O	O	O	O	O	O	O	O	O	O
Spotting	O	O	O	O	O	O	O	O	O	O	O	O	O	O	O	O	O	O	O	O
Dry	O	O	O	O	O	O	O	O	O	O	O	O	O	O	O	O	O	O	O	O
Creamy	O	O	O	O	O	O	O	O	O	O	O	O	O	O	O	O	O	O	O	O
Slippery	O	O	O	O	O	O	O	O	O	O	O	O	O	O	O	O	O	O	O	O

CATEGORIES

CYCLE DAY	1	2	3	4	5	6	7	8	9	10	11	12	13	14	15	16	17	18	19	20
1 Comfort	O	O	O	O	O	O	O	O	O	O	O	O	O	O	O	O	O	O	O	O
2	O	O	O	O	O	O	O	O	O	O	O	O	O	O	O	O	O	O	O	O
3	O	O	O	O	O	O	O	O	O	O	O	O	O	O	O	O	O	O	O	O
4	O	O	O	O	O	O	O	O	O	O	O	O	O	O	O	O	O	O	O	O
5	O	O	O	O	O	O	O	O	O	O	O	O	O	O	O	O	O	O	O	O
5	O	O	O	O	O	O	O	O	O	O	O	O	O	O	O	O	O	O	O	O
5	O	O	O	O	O	O	O	O	O	O	O	O	O	O	O	O	O	O	O	O
6	O	O	O	O	O	O	O	O	O	O	O	O	O	O	O	O	O	O	O	O
6	O	O	O	O	O	O	O	O	O	O	O	O	O	O	O	O	O	O	O	O

BASAL BODY TEMPERATURES

| 21 | 22 | 23 | 24 | 25 | 26 | 27 | 28 | 29 | 30 | 31 | 32 | 33 | 34 | 35 | 36 | 37 | 38 | 39 | 40 | CYCLE DAY |

Higher Baseline BBT — _____ F/C

9 8 7 6 5 4 3 2 1 0 (rows of circled numbers for each cycle day)

Lower Baseline BBT — _____ F/C

9 8 7 6 5 4 3 2 1 0 (rows of circled numbers for each cycle day)

BODY FLUIDS

21	22	23	24	25	26	27	28	29	30	31	32	33	34	35	36	37	38	39	40	CYCLE DAY
○	○	○	○	○	○	○	○	○	○	○	○	○	○	○	○	○	○	○	○	Bleeding
○	○	○	○	○	○	○	○	○	○	○	○	○	○	○	○	○	○	○	○	Spotting
○	○	○	○	○	○	○	○	○	○	○	○	○	○	○	○	○	○	○	○	Dry
○	○	○	○	○	○	○	○	○	○	○	○	○	○	○	○	○	○	○	○	Creamy
○	○	○	○	○	○	○	○	○	○	○	○	○	○	○	○	○	○	○	○	Slippery

CATEGORIES

21	22	23	24	25	26	27	28	29	30	31	32	33	34	35	36	37	38	39	40	CYCLE DAY	
○	○	○	○	○	○	○	○	○	○	○	○	○	○	○	○	○	○	○	○	Comfort	1
○	○	○	○	○	○	○	○	○	○	○	○	○	○	○	○	○	○	○	○		2
○	○	○	○	○	○	○	○	○	○	○	○	○	○	○	○	○	○	○	○		3
○	○	○	○	○	○	○	○	○	○	○	○	○	○	○	○	○	○	○	○		4
○	○	○	○	○	○	○	○	○	○	○	○	○	○	○	○	○	○	○	○		
○	○	○	○	○	○	○	○	○	○	○	○	○	○	○	○	○	○	○	○		
○	○	○	○	○	○	○	○	○	○	○	○	○	○	○	○	○	○	○	○		5
○	○	○	○	○	○	○	○	○	○	○	○	○	○	○	○	○	○	○	○		
○	○	○	○	○	○	○	○	○	○	○	○	○	○	○	○	○	○	○	○		
○	○	○	○	○	○	○	○	○	○	○	○	○	○	○	○	○	○	○	○		6

CYCLE REVIEW

Analyze your last cycle and prepare for your next

BASELINE INSIGHTS

BASAL BODY TEMPERATURE

Can you identify a significant and sustained temperature increase and the day it began? ○ Yes ○ No ○ I'm not sure

_____

_____

BODY FLUID

Can you identify which day you experienced the most slippery fluid for this last cycle? ○ Yes ○ No ○ I'm not sure

_____

_____

Could you easily differentiate bleeding and spotting for this last cycle? ○ Yes ○ No ○ I'm not sure

_____

_____

Did you notice other body fluids during this last cycle? ○ Yes ○ No ○ I'm not sure

_____

_____

PATTERNS

Starting with comfort, review your list of categories tracked last cycle.

Were you able to identify feelings of *comfort* during your last cycle? ○ Yes ○ No ○ I'm not sure

Did you notice a change in how you felt on the days when comfort was present? ○ Yes ○ No ○ I'm not sure

Write your other categories from last cycle below and use symbols for "More," "Less," and "I'm not sure."

(+) More   (−) Less   (?) I'm not sure

Are categories more or less present during the bleeding phase of your cycle?

_____ ○ _____ ○ _____ ○ _____ ○ _____ ○

What categories seem to be more or less present when you notice slippery cervical fluid?

_____ ○ _____ ○ _____ ○ _____ ○ _____ ○

What categories seem to be more or less present right before your next bleeding phase?

_____ ○ _____ ○ _____ ○ _____ ○ _____ ○

GENERAL MOOD

Are you getting what you need out of tracking?

○ Yes, this is totally working   ○ I think I'm onto something   ○ Not yet, finding more support feels like a good next step

What patterns are you curious about for your next cycle?

_____

Which categories appear unrelated to phases of your cycle?

_____

CATEGORY INSIGHTS

Write your categories from last cycle below and use symbols for keeping, refining, and dropping those descriptions.

Do any categories need a bit of refining?   What categories are you going to track next cycle?

(✔) Keep   (→) Refine   (X) Drop

_____   ○   _____

_____   ○   _____

_____   ○   _____

_____   ○   _____

_____   ○   _____

CYCLE PREVIEW

What are your 3 goals for this next cycle of tracking?

_____   _____   _____

What will you do differently for your next cycle?

_____

_____

What are 2 ways you can introduce comfort, safety, and/or pleasure into your cycle?

_____   _____

What are 2 ways you can make cycle tracking easier for you?

_____   _____

CYCLE

MONTH _____ DATE ___ __ __ __ __ __ __ __ __ __ __ __ __ __ __ __ __ __ __ __

BASAL BODY TEMPERATURES

CYCLE DAY 1 2 3 4 5 6 7 8 9 10 11 12 13 14 15 16 17 18 19 20

_____ F/C — Higher Baseline BBT

Rows (for each cycle day column): 9 8 7 6 5 4 3 2 1 0

_____ F/C — Lower Baseline BBT

Rows (for each cycle day column): 9 8 7 6 5 4 3 2 1 0

BODY FLUIDS

CYCLE DAY 1 2 3 4 5 6 7 8 9 10 11 12 13 14 15 16 17 18 19 20

Bleeding	○	○	○	○	○	○	○	○	○	○	○	○	○	○	○	○	○	○	○	○
Spotting	○	○	○	○	○	○	○	○	○	○	○	○	○	○	○	○	○	○	○	○
Dry	○	○	○	○	○	○	○	○	○	○	○	○	○	○	○	○	○	○	○	○
Creamy	○	○	○	○	○	○	○	○	○	○	○	○	○	○	○	○	○	○	○	○
Slippery	○	○	○	○	○	○	○	○	○	○	○	○	○	○	○	○	○	○	○	○

CATEGORIES

CYCLE DAY 1 2 3 4 5 6 7 8 9 10 11 12 13 14 15 16 17 18 19 20

1 Comfort	○	○	○	○	○	○	○	○	○	○	○	○	○	○	○	○	○	○	○	○
2	○	○	○	○	○	○	○	○	○	○	○	○	○	○	○	○	○	○	○	○
3	○	○	○	○	○	○	○	○	○	○	○	○	○	○	○	○	○	○	○	○
4	○	○	○	○	○	○	○	○	○	○	○	○	○	○	○	○	○	○	○	○
5	○	○	○	○	○	○	○	○	○	○	○	○	○	○	○	○	○	○	○	○
5	○	○	○	○	○	○	○	○	○	○	○	○	○	○	○	○	○	○	○	○
5	○	○	○	○	○	○	○	○	○	○	○	○	○	○	○	○	○	○	○	○
6	○	○	○	○	○	○	○	○	○	○	○	○	○	○	○	○	○	○	○	○
6	○	○	○	○	○	○	○	○	○	○	○	○	○	○	○	○	○	○	○	○
6	○	○	○	○	○	○	○	○	○	○	○	○	○	○	○	○	○	○	○	○

BASAL BODY TEMPERATURES

| 21 | 22 | 23 | 24 | 25 | 26 | 27 | 28 | 29 | 30 | 31 | 32 | 33 | 34 | 35 | 36 | 37 | 38 | 39 | 40 | CYCLE DAY |

Higher Baseline BBT _____ F/C

9 9 9 9 9 9 9 9 9 9 9 9 9 9 9 9 9 9 9 9
8 8 8 8 8 8 8 8 8 8 8 8 8 8 8 8 8 8 8 8
7 7 7 7 7 7 7 7 7 7 7 7 7 7 7 7 7 7 7 7
6 6 6 6 6 6 6 6 6 6 6 6 6 6 6 6 6 6 6 6
5 5 5 5 5 5 5 5 5 5 5 5 5 5 5 5 5 5 5 5
4 4 4 4 4 4 4 4 4 4 4 4 4 4 4 4 4 4 4 4
3 3 3 3 3 3 3 3 3 3 3 3 3 3 3 3 3 3 3 3
2 2 2 2 2 2 2 2 2 2 2 2 2 2 2 2 2 2 2 2
1 1 1 1 1 1 1 1 1 1 1 1 1 1 1 1 1 1 1 1
0 0 0 0 0 0 0 0 0 0 0 0 0 0 0 0 0 0 0 0

Lower Baseline BBT _____ F/C

9 9 9 9 9 9 9 9 9 9 9 9 9 9 9 9 9 9 9 9
8 8 8 8 8 8 8 8 8 8 8 8 8 8 8 8 8 8 8 8
7 7 7 7 7 7 7 7 7 7 7 7 7 7 7 7 7 7 7 7
6 6 6 6 6 6 6 6 6 6 6 6 6 6 6 6 6 6 6 6
5 5 5 5 5 5 5 5 5 5 5 5 5 5 5 5 5 5 5 5
4 4 4 4 4 4 4 4 4 4 4 4 4 4 4 4 4 4 4 4
3 3 3 3 3 3 3 3 3 3 3 3 3 3 3 3 3 3 3 3
2 2 2 2 2 2 2 2 2 2 2 2 2 2 2 2 2 2 2 2
1 1 1 1 1 1 1 1 1 1 1 1 1 1 1 1 1 1 1 1
0 0 0 0 0 0 0 0 0 0 0 0 0 0 0 0 0 0 0 0

BODY FLUIDS

21	22	23	24	25	26	27	28	29	30	31	32	33	34	35	36	37	38	39	40	CYCLE DAY
O	O	O	O	O	O	O	O	O	O	O	O	O	O	O	O	O	O	O	O	Bleeding
O	O	O	O	O	O	O	O	O	O	O	O	O	O	O	O	O	O	O	O	Spotting
O	O	O	O	O	O	O	O	O	O	O	O	O	O	O	O	O	O	O	O	Dry
O	O	O	O	O	O	O	O	O	O	O	O	O	O	O	O	O	O	O	O	Creamy
O	O	O	O	O	O	O	O	O	O	O	O	O	O	O	O	O	O	O	O	Slippery

CATEGORIES

21	22	23	24	25	26	27	28	29	30	31	32	33	34	35	36	37	38	39	40	CYCLE DAY	
O	O	O	O	O	O	O	O	O	O	O	O	O	O	O	O	O	O	O	O	Comfort	1
O	O	O	O	O	O	O	O	O	O	O	O	O	O	O	O	O	O	O	O		2
O	O	O	O	O	O	O	O	O	O	O	O	O	O	O	O	O	O	O	O		3
O	O	O	O	O	O	O	O	O	O	O	O	O	O	O	O	O	O	O	O		4
O	O	O	O	O	O	O	O	O	O	O	O	O	O	O	O	O	O	O	O		
O	O	O	O	O	O	O	O	O	O	O	O	O	O	O	O	O	O	O	O		
O	O	O	O	O	O	O	O	O	O	O	O	O	O	O	O	O	O	O	O		5
O	O	O	O	O	O	O	O	O	O	O	O	O	O	O	O	O	O	O	O		
O	O	O	O	O	O	O	O	O	O	O	O	O	O	O	O	O	O	O	O		
O	O	O	O	O	O	O	O	O	O	O	O	O	O	O	O	O	O	O	O		6

CYCLE REVIEW

Analyze your last cycle and prepare for your next

BASELINE INSIGHTS

BASAL BODY TEMPERATURE

Can you identify a significant and sustained temperature increase and the day it began? ○ Yes ○ No ○ I'm not sure

_____

_____

BODY FLUID

Can you identify which day you experienced the most slippery fluid for this last cycle? ○ Yes ○ No ○ I'm not sure

_____

_____

Could you easily differentiate bleeding and spotting for this last cycle? ○ Yes ○ No ○ I'm not sure

_____

_____

Did you notice other body fluids during this last cycle? ○ Yes ○ No ○ I'm not sure

_____

_____

PATTERNS

Starting with comfort, review your list of categories tracked last cycle.

Were you able to identify feelings of *comfort* during your last cycle? ○ Yes ○ No ○ I'm not sure

Did you notice a change in how you felt on the days when comfort was present? ○ Yes ○ No ○ I'm not sure

Write your other categories from last cycle below and use symbols for "More," "Less," and "I'm not sure."

(+) More   (−) Less   (?) I'm not sure

Are categories more or less present during the bleeding phase of your cycle?

_____○_____○_____○_____○_____○

What categories seem to be more or less present when you notice slippery cervical fluid?

_____○_____○_____○_____○_____○

What categories seem to be more or less present right before your next bleeding phase?

_____○_____○_____○_____○_____○

GENERAL MOOD

Are you getting what you need out of tracking?

○ Yes, this is totally working   ○ I think I'm onto something   ○ Not yet, finding more support feels like a good next step

What patterns are you curious about for your next cycle?

_____

Which categories appear unrelated to phases of your cycle?

_____

CATEGORY INSIGHTS

Write your categories from last cycle below and use symbols for keeping, refining, and dropping those descriptions.

Do any categories need a bit of refining?   What categories are you going to track next cycle?

(✔) Keep   (→) Refine   (✗) Drop

_____   ○   _____
_____   ○   _____
_____   ○   _____
_____   ○   _____
_____   ○   _____

CYCLE PREVIEW

What are your 3 goals for this next cycle of tracking?

_____   _____   _____

What will you do differently for your next cycle?

_____

What are 2 ways you can introduce comfort, safety, and/or pleasure into your cycle?

_____   _____

What are 2 ways you can make cycle tracking easier for you?

_____   _____

CYCLE

MONTH _____ DATE ___ __ __ ___ __ __ ___ __ __

BASAL BODY TEMPERATURES

Higher Baseline BBT — _____ F/C

CYCLE DAY	1	2	3	4	5	6	7	8	9	10	11	12	13	14	15	16	17	18	19	20

(Temperature grid, values 9 down to 0 for each cycle day)

Lower Baseline BBT — _____ F/C

(Temperature grid, values 9 down to 0 for each cycle day)

BODY FLUIDS

CYCLE DAY	1	2	3	4	5	6	7	8	9	10	11	12	13	14	15	16	17	18	19	20
Bleeding	O	O	O	O	O	O	O	O	O	O	O	O	O	O	O	O	O	O	O	O
Spotting	O	O	O	O	O	O	O	O	O	O	O	O	O	O	O	O	O	O	O	O
Dry	O	O	O	O	O	O	O	O	O	O	O	O	O	O	O	O	O	O	O	O
Creamy	O	O	O	O	O	O	O	O	O	O	O	O	O	O	O	O	O	O	O	O
Slippery	O	O	O	O	O	O	O	O	O	O	O	O	O	O	O	O	O	O	O	O

CATEGORIES

CYCLE DAY	1	2	3	4	5	6	7	8	9	10	11	12	13	14	15	16	17	18	19	20
1 Comfort	O	O	O	O	O	O	O	O	O	O	O	O	O	O	O	O	O	O	O	O
2	O	O	O	O	O	O	O	O	O	O	O	O	O	O	O	O	O	O	O	O
3	O	O	O	O	O	O	O	O	O	O	O	O	O	O	O	O	O	O	O	O
4	O	O	O	O	O	O	O	O	O	O	O	O	O	O	O	O	O	O	O	O
5	O	O	O	O	O	O	O	O	O	O	O	O	O	O	O	O	O	O	O	O
	O	O	O	O	O	O	O	O	O	O	O	O	O	O	O	O	O	O	O	O
	O	O	O	O	O	O	O	O	O	O	O	O	O	O	O	O	O	O	O	O
6	O	O	O	O	O	O	O	O	O	O	O	O	O	O	O	O	O	O	O	O
	O	O	O	O	O	O	O	O	O	O	O	O	O	O	O	O	O	O	O	O
	O	O	O	O	O	O	O	O	O	O	O	O	O	O	O	O	O	O	O	O

BASAL BODY TEMPERATURES

| 21 | 22 | 23 | 24 | 25 | 26 | 27 | 28 | 29 | 30 | 31 | 32 | 33 | 34 | 35 | 36 | 37 | 38 | 39 | 40 | CYCLE DAY |

Higher Baseline BBT

Rows (each column 21–40): 9 8 7 6 5 4 3 2 1 0

_____ F/C

Lower Baseline BBT

Rows (each column 21–40): 9 8 7 6 5 4 3 2 1 0

_____ F/C

BODY FLUIDS

21	22	23	24	25	26	27	28	29	30	31	32	33	34	35	36	37	38	39	40	CYCLE DAY
○	○	○	○	○	○	○	○	○	○	○	○	○	○	○	○	○	○	○	○	Bleeding
○	○	○	○	○	○	○	○	○	○	○	○	○	○	○	○	○	○	○	○	Spotting
○	○	○	○	○	○	○	○	○	○	○	○	○	○	○	○	○	○	○	○	Dry
○	○	○	○	○	○	○	○	○	○	○	○	○	○	○	○	○	○	○	○	Creamy
○	○	○	○	○	○	○	○	○	○	○	○	○	○	○	○	○	○	○	○	Slippery

CATEGORIES

21	22	23	24	25	26	27	28	29	30	31	32	33	34	35	36	37	38	39	40	CYCLE DAY	
○	○	○	○	○	○	○	○	○	○	○	○	○	○	○	○	○	○	○	○	Comfort	1
○	○	○	○	○	○	○	○	○	○	○	○	○	○	○	○	○	○	○	○		2
○	○	○	○	○	○	○	○	○	○	○	○	○	○	○	○	○	○	○	○		3
○	○	○	○	○	○	○	○	○	○	○	○	○	○	○	○	○	○	○	○		4
○	○	○	○	○	○	○	○	○	○	○	○	○	○	○	○	○	○	○	○		
○	○	○	○	○	○	○	○	○	○	○	○	○	○	○	○	○	○	○	○		5
○	○	○	○	○	○	○	○	○	○	○	○	○	○	○	○	○	○	○	○		
○	○	○	○	○	○	○	○	○	○	○	○	○	○	○	○	○	○	○	○		
○	○	○	○	○	○	○	○	○	○	○	○	○	○	○	○	○	○	○	○		6

CYCLE REVIEW
Analyze your last cycle and prepare for your next

BASELINE INSIGHTS

BASAL BODY TEMPERATURE

Can you identify a significant and sustained temperature increase and the day it began? ○ Yes ○ No ○ I'm not sure

_____

_____

BODY FLUID

Can you identify which day you experienced the most slippery fluid for this last cycle? ○ Yes ○ No ○ I'm not sure

_____

_____

Could you easily differentiate bleeding and spotting for this last cycle? ○ Yes ○ No ○ I'm not sure

_____

_____

Did you notice other body fluids during this last cycle? ○ Yes ○ No ○ I'm not sure

_____

_____

PATTERNS

Starting with comfort, review your list of categories tracked last cycle.

Were you able to identify feelings of *comfort* during your last cycle? ○ Yes ○ No ○ I'm not sure

Did you notice a change in how you felt on the days when comfort was present? ○ Yes ○ No ○ I'm not sure

Write your other categories from last cycle below and use symbols for "More," "Less," and "I'm not sure."

(+) More   (−) Less   (?) I'm not sure

Are categories more or less present during the bleeding phase of your cycle?

_____○_____○_____○_____○_____○

What categories seem to be more or less present when you notice slippery cervical fluid?

_____○_____○_____○_____○_____○

What categories seem to be more or less present right before your next bleeding phase?

_____○_____○_____○_____○_____○

GENERAL MOOD

Are you getting what you need out of tracking?

○ Yes, this is totally working ○ I think I'm onto something ○ Not yet, finding more support feels like a good next step

What patterns are you curious about for your next cycle?

_____

Which categories appear unrelated to phases of your cycle?

_____

CATEGORY INSIGHTS

Write your categories from last cycle below and use symbols for keeping, refining, and dropping those descriptions.

Do any categories need a bit of refining?   What categories are you going to track next cycle?

✔ Keep   → Refine   ✗ Drop

_____   ○   _____
_____   ○   _____
_____   ○   _____
_____   ○   _____
_____   ○   _____

CYCLE PREVIEW

What are your 3 goals for this next cycle of tracking?

_____   _____   _____

What will you do differently for your next cycle?

_____

_____

What are 2 ways you can introduce comfort, safety, and/or pleasure into your cycle?

_____   _____

What are 2 ways you can make cycle tracking easier for you?

_____   _____

CYCLE

MONTH _____ DATE ___ ___ ___ ___ ___ ___ ___ ___ ___ ___ ___ ___ ___ ___ ___ ___ ___ ___ ___

BASAL BODY TEMPERATURES

CYCLE DAY	1	2	3	4	5	6	7	8	9	10	11	12	13	14	15	16	17	18	19	20

_____ F/C — Higher Baseline BBT

(Grid of numbered circles 9 through 0 for each cycle day 1–20)

_____ F/C — Lower Baseline BBT

(Grid of numbered circles 9 through 0 for each cycle day 1–20)

BODY FLUIDS

CYCLE DAY	1	2	3	4	5	6	7	8	9	10	11	12	13	14	15	16	17	18	19	20
Bleeding	O	O	O	O	O	O	O	O	O	O	O	O	O	O	O	O	O	O	O	O
Spotting	O	O	O	O	O	O	O	O	O	O	O	O	O	O	O	O	O	O	O	O
Dry	O	O	O	O	O	O	O	O	O	O	O	O	O	O	O	O	O	O	O	O
Creamy	O	O	O	O	O	O	O	O	O	O	O	O	O	O	O	O	O	O	O	O
Slippery	O	O	O	O	O	O	O	O	O	O	O	O	O	O	O	O	O	O	O	O

CATEGORIES

CYCLE DAY	1	2	3	4	5	6	7	8	9	10	11	12	13	14	15	16	17	18	19	20
1 Comfort	O	O	O	O	O	O	O	O	O	O	O	O	O	O	O	O	O	O	O	O
2	O	O	O	O	O	O	O	O	O	O	O	O	O	O	O	O	O	O	O	O
3	O	O	O	O	O	O	O	O	O	O	O	O	O	O	O	O	O	O	O	O
4	O	O	O	O	O	O	O	O	O	O	O	O	O	O	O	O	O	O	O	O
5	O	O	O	O	O	O	O	O	O	O	O	O	O	O	O	O	O	O	O	O
6	O	O	O	O	O	O	O	O	O	O	O	O	O	O	O	O	O	O	O	O

BASAL BODY TEMPERATURES

| CYCLE DAY | 21 | 22 | 23 | 24 | 25 | 26 | 27 | 28 | 29 | 30 | 31 | 32 | 33 | 34 | 35 | 36 | 37 | 38 | 39 | 40 |

Higher Baseline BBT _____ F/C

Temperature grid (values 9 through 0 for each cycle day 21–40)

Lower Baseline BBT _____ F/C

Temperature grid (values 9 through 0 for each cycle day 21–40)

BODY FLUIDS

CYCLE DAY	21	22	23	24	25	26	27	28	29	30	31	32	33	34	35	36	37	38	39	40	
	○	○	○	○	○	○	○	○	○	○	○	○	○	○	○	○	○	○	○	○	Bleeding
	○	○	○	○	○	○	○	○	○	○	○	○	○	○	○	○	○	○	○	○	Spotting
	○	○	○	○	○	○	○	○	○	○	○	○	○	○	○	○	○	○	○	○	Dry
	○	○	○	○	○	○	○	○	○	○	○	○	○	○	○	○	○	○	○	○	Creamy
	○	○	○	○	○	○	○	○	○	○	○	○	○	○	○	○	○	○	○	○	Slippery

CATEGORIES

CYCLE DAY	21	22	23	24	25	26	27	28	29	30	31	32	33	34	35	36	37	38	39	40		
	○	○	○	○	○	○	○	○	○	○	○	○	○	○	○	○	○	○	○	○	Comfort	1
	○	○	○	○	○	○	○	○	○	○	○	○	○	○	○	○	○	○	○	○		2
	○	○	○	○	○	○	○	○	○	○	○	○	○	○	○	○	○	○	○	○		3
	○	○	○	○	○	○	○	○	○	○	○	○	○	○	○	○	○	○	○	○		4
	○	○	○	○	○	○	○	○	○	○	○	○	○	○	○	○	○	○	○			
	○	○	○	○	○	○	○	○	○	○	○	○	○	○	○	○	○	○	○			
	○	○	○	○	○	○	○	○	○	○	○	○	○	○	○	○	○	○	○			5
	○	○	○	○	○	○	○	○	○	○	○	○	○	○	○	○	○	○	○			
	○	○	○	○	○	○	○	○	○	○	○	○	○	○	○	○	○	○	○			
	○	○	○	○	○	○	○	○	○	○	○	○	○	○	○	○	○	○	○			6

CYCLE REVIEW

Analyze your last cycle and prepare for your next

BASELINE INSIGHTS

BASAL BODY TEMPERATURE

Can you identify a significant and sustained temperature increase and the day it began?   ○ Yes ○ No ○ I'm not sure

_____

_____

BODY FLUID

Can you identify which day you experienced the most slippery fluid for this last cycle?   ○ Yes ○ No ○ I'm not sure

_____

_____

Could you easily differentiate bleeding and spotting for this last cycle?   ○ Yes ○ No ○ I'm not sure

_____

_____

Did you notice other body fluids during this last cycle?   ○ Yes ○ No ○ I'm not sure

_____

_____

PATTERNS

Starting with comfort, review your list of categories tracked last cycle.

Were you able to identify feelings of *comfort* during your last cycle?   ○ Yes ○ No ○ I'm not sure

Did you notice a change in how you felt on the days when comfort was present?   ○ Yes ○ No ○ I'm not sure

Write your other categories from last cycle below and use symbols for "More," "Less," and "I'm not sure."

(+) More   (−) Less   (?) I'm not sure

Are categories more or less present during the bleeding phase of your cycle?

___○___ ___○___ ___○___ ___○___ ___○___

What categories seem to be more or less present when you notice slippery cervical fluid?

___○___ ___○___ ___○___ ___○___ ___○___

What categories seem to be more or less present right before your next bleeding phase?

___○___ ___○___ ___○___ ___○___ ___○___

GENERAL MOOD

Are you getting what you need out of tracking?

○ Yes, this is totally working   ○ I think I'm onto something   ○ Not yet, finding more support feels like a good next step

What patterns are you curious about for your next cycle?

_____

Which categories appear unrelated to phases of your cycle?

_____

CATEGORY INSIGHTS

Write your categories from last cycle below and use symbols for keeping, refining, and dropping those descriptions.

Do any categories need a bit of refining?   What categories are you going to track next cycle?

✔ Keep   → Refine   ✗ Drop

_____   ○   _____
_____   ○   _____
_____   ○   _____
_____   ○   _____
_____   ○   _____

CYCLE PREVIEW

What are your 3 goals for this next cycle of tracking?

_____   _____   _____

What will you do differently for your next cycle?

_____

_____

What are 2 ways you can introduce comfort, safety, and/or pleasure into your cycle?

_____   _____

What are 2 ways you can make cycle tracking easier for you?

_____   _____

CYCLE

MONTH ____________ DATE ___

BASAL BODY TEMPERATURES

____ F/C — Higher Baseline BBT

CYCLE DAY	1	2	3	4	5	6	7	8	9	10	11	12	13	14	15	16	17	18	19	20
	9	9	9	9	9	9	9	9	9	9	9	9	9	9	9	9	9	9	9	9
	8	8	8	8	8	8	8	8	8	8	8	8	8	8	8	8	8	8	8	8
	7	7	7	7	7	7	7	7	7	7	7	7	7	7	7	7	7	7	7	7
	6	6	6	6	6	6	6	6	6	6	6	6	6	6	6	6	6	6	6	6
	5	5	5	5	5	5	5	5	5	5	5	5	5	5	5	5	5	5	5	5
	4	4	4	4	4	4	4	4	4	4	4	4	4	4	4	4	4	4	4	4
	3	3	3	3	3	3	3	3	3	3	3	3	3	3	3	3	3	3	3	3
	2	2	2	2	2	2	2	2	2	2	2	2	2	2	2	2	2	2	2	2
	1	1	1	1	1	1	1	1	1	1	1	1	1	1	1	1	1	1	1	1
	0	0	0	0	0	0	0	0	0	0	0	0	0	0	0	0	0	0	0	0

____ F/C — Lower Baseline BBT

	9	9	9	9	9	9	9	9	9	9	9	9	9	9	9	9	9	9	9	9
	8	8	8	8	8	8	8	8	8	8	8	8	8	8	8	8	8	8	8	8
	7	7	7	7	7	7	7	7	7	7	7	7	7	7	7	7	7	7	7	7
	6	6	6	6	6	6	6	6	6	6	6	6	6	6	6	6	6	6	6	6
	5	5	5	5	5	5	5	5	5	5	5	5	5	5	5	5	5	5	5	5
	4	4	4	4	4	4	4	4	4	4	4	4	4	4	4	4	4	4	4	4
	3	3	3	3	3	3	3	3	3	3	3	3	3	3	3	3	3	3	3	3
	2	2	2	2	2	2	2	2	2	2	2	2	2	2	2	2	2	2	2	2
	1	1	1	1	1	1	1	1	1	1	1	1	1	1	1	1	1	1	1	1
	0	0	0	0	0	0	0	0	0	0	0	0	0	0	0	0	0	0	0	0

BODY FLUIDS

CYCLE DAY	1	2	3	4	5	6	7	8	9	10	11	12	13	14	15	16	17	18	19	20
Bleeding	O	O	O	O	O	O	O	O	O	O	O	O	O	O	O	O	O	O	O	O
Spotting	O	O	O	O	O	O	O	O	O	O	O	O	O	O	O	O	O	O	O	O
Dry	O	O	O	O	O	O	O	O	O	O	O	O	O	O	O	O	O	O	O	O
Creamy	O	O	O	O	O	O	O	O	O	O	O	O	O	O	O	O	O	O	O	O
Slippery	O	O	O	O	O	O	O	O	O	O	O	O	O	O	O	O	O	O	O	O

CATEGORIES

CYCLE DAY	1	2	3	4	5	6	7	8	9	10	11	12	13	14	15	16	17	18	19	20
1 Comfort	O	O	O	O	O	O	O	O	O	O	O	O	O	O	O	O	O	O	O	O
2	O	O	O	O	O	O	O	O	O	O	O	O	O	O	O	O	O	O	O	O
3	O	O	O	O	O	O	O	O	O	O	O	O	O	O	O	O	O	O	O	O
4	O	O	O	O	O	O	O	O	O	O	O	O	O	O	O	O	O	O	O	O
	O	O	O	O	O	O	O	O	O	O	O	O	O	O	O	O	O	O	O	O
	O	O	O	O	O	O	O	O	O	O	O	O	O	O	O	O	O	O	O	O
5	O	O	O	O	O	O	O	O	O	O	O	O	O	O	O	O	O	O	O	O
	O	O	O	O	O	O	O	O	O	O	O	O	O	O	O	O	O	O	O	O
	O	O	O	O	O	O	O	O	O	O	O	O	O	O	O	O	O	O	O	O
6	O	O	O	O	O	O	O	O	O	O	O	O	O	O	O	O	O	O	O	O

BASAL BODY TEMPERATURES

21	22	23	24	25	26	27	28	29	30	31	32	33	34	35	36	37	38	39	40	CYCLE DAY

Higher Baseline BBT — _____ F/C

Rows (top to bottom): 9 8 7 6 5 4 3 2 1 0 (for each cycle day 21–40)

Lower Baseline BBT — _____ F/C

Rows (top to bottom): 9 8 7 6 5 4 3 2 1 0 (for each cycle day 21–40)

BODY FLUIDS

21	22	23	24	25	26	27	28	29	30	31	32	33	34	35	36	37	38	39	40	CYCLE DAY
O	O	O	O	O	O	O	O	O	O	O	O	O	O	O	O	O	O	O	O	Bleeding
O	O	O	O	O	O	O	O	O	O	O	O	O	O	O	O	O	O	O	O	Spotting
O	O	O	O	O	O	O	O	O	O	O	O	O	O	O	O	O	O	O	O	Dry
O	O	O	O	O	O	O	O	O	O	O	O	O	O	O	O	O	O	O	O	Creamy
O	O	O	O	O	O	O	O	O	O	O	O	O	O	O	O	O	O	O	O	Slippery

CATEGORIES

21	22	23	24	25	26	27	28	29	30	31	32	33	34	35	36	37	38	39	40	CYCLE DAY	
O	O	O	O	O	O	O	O	O	O	O	O	O	O	O	O	O	O	O	O	Comfort	1
O	O	O	O	O	O	O	O	O	O	O	O	O	O	O	O	O	O	O	O		2
O	O	O	O	O	O	O	O	O	O	O	O	O	O	O	O	O	O	O	O		3
O	O	O	O	O	O	O	O	O	O	O	O	O	O	O	O	O	O	O	O		4
O	O	O	O	O	O	O	O	O	O	O	O	O	O	O	O	O	O	O	O		
O	O	O	O	O	O	O	O	O	O	O	O	O	O	O	O	O	O	O	O		5
O	O	O	O	O	O	O	O	O	O	O	O	O	O	O	O	O	O	O	O		
O	O	O	O	O	O	O	O	O	O	O	O	O	O	O	O	O	O	O	O		6

CYCLE REVIEW

Analyze your last cycle and prepare for your next

BASELINE INSIGHTS

BASAL BODY TEMPERATURE

Can you identify a significant and sustained temperature increase and the day it began? ○ Yes ○ No ○ I'm not sure

_____

_____

BODY FLUID

Can you identify which day you experienced the most slippery fluid for this last cycle?   ○ Yes ○ No ○ I'm not sure

_____

_____

Could you easily differentiate bleeding and spotting for this last cycle?   ○ Yes ○ No ○ I'm not sure

_____

_____

Did you notice other body fluids during this last cycle?   ○ Yes ○ No ○ I'm not sure

_____

_____

PATTERNS

*Starting with **comfort**, review your list of categories tracked last cycle.*

Were you able to identify feelings of *comfort* during your last cycle?   ○ Yes ○ No ○ I'm not sure

Did you notice a change in how you felt on the days when comfort was present?   ○ Yes ○ No ○ I'm not sure

Write your other categories from last cycle below and use symbols for "More," "Less," and "I'm not sure."

(+) More   (−) Less   (?) I'm not sure

Are categories more or less present during the bleeding phase of your cycle?

____○ ____○ ____○ ____○ ____○

What categories seem to be more or less present when you notice slippery cervical fluid?

____○ ____○ ____○ ____○ ____○

What categories seem to be more or less present right before your next bleeding phase?

____○ ____○ ____○ ____○ ____○

GENERAL MOOD

Are you getting what you need out of tracking?

○ Yes, this is totally working ○ I think I'm onto something ○ Not yet, finding more support feels like a good next step

What patterns are you curious about for your next cycle?

_____

Which categories appear unrelated to phases of your cycle?

_____

CATEGORY INSIGHTS

Write your categories from last cycle below and use symbols for keeping, refining, and dropping those descriptions.

Do any categories need a bit of refining?   What categories are you going to track next cycle?

✔ Keep   → Refine   ✗ Drop

_____   ○   _____

_____   ○   _____

_____   ○   _____

_____   ○   _____

_____   ○

CYCLE PREVIEW

What are your 3 goals for this next cycle of tracking?

_____   _____   _____

What will you do differently for your next cycle?

_____

_____

What are 2 ways you can introduce comfort, safety, and/or pleasure into your cycle?

_____   _____

What are 2 ways you can make cycle tracking easier for you?

_____   _____

13.

Your Cycle Patterns

So you've gathered all this critical information. How do we understand it?

With our clients, we start with a simple chart analysis. To recognize patterns within your cycle, note where your categories fall on your chart in comparison to where your biomarkers fall.

If categories show up at similar points of each cycle, exploring the hormonal significance can aid you in understanding the sensations' regular entrances into your life. You may find that expecting a sensation's arrival each cycle is helpful. Or maybe there are ways you learn to prep for that sensation that align with your overall goals. You may decide to take active steps toward a more intensive intervention.

HOW TO INTERPRET BIOMARKER DATA

Basal Body Temperature (BBT)

When you review your last cycle's recorded daily temperatures, you will notice ups and downs.

A sustained temperature increase can mean:
    An increase in your progesterone levels
    You shifted from your follicular to luteal cycle phase

A sustained temperature decrease can mean:
    A decrease in your progesterone levels
    You shifted from your luteal to follicular phase

Minimal temperature increases (less than 0.3°C or 0.5°F) can mean:
    Low progesterone levels

A sudden significant dip in temperature followed by a sudden sustained peak in temperature can mean:
    You may have been nearing ovulation

Some experiences that could lead to a shift in temperature should be considered outliers. The most common causes of these nonhormonal temperature changes we see are illness, alcohol, fever, and the temperature of your environment. For example, falling asleep with the heat on high and extra blankets might lead to a slight increase in body temperature unrelated to hormonal shifts.

Body Fluid

When you observe your body fluid tracking data, you will notice shifts between types and consistency of your fluids.

Bleeding can mean:

A decrease in your progesterone levels

An increase in your estrogen levels

You are in your menstrual phase

Clear and slippery egg-white fluid can mean:

An increase in your LH levels

A sudden peak and fall of your estrogen levels

An impending increase in your progesterone levels

An indication of your ovulatory phase (some people may also experience this body fluid *without* ovulating)

Shifting from your follicular phase to your luteal phase

Creamy and lotionlike fluid can mean:

Transitioning into or away from your ovulatory phase

Dryness can mean:

Transitioning into or away from your bleeding phase

Let's take a peek at some charts to see how we can triangulate data to understand patterns. Use any lines, circles, arrows, zigzags, or punctuation marks you'd like on your charts to identify patterns and phases. Here are a few examples of charts in use.

CYCLE

This temperature is circled because it stands out from the rest of Nasreen's temperatures, and it may be an outlier. In retrospect, Nasreen recalls she had a particularly bad night of insomnia on May 1st. That sleep disruption can alter a BBT. It's okay to have an outlier, so Nasreen chooses to simply disregard this one.

MONTH

| 28 | 29 | 30 | 1 | 2 | 3 | 4 | 5 | 6 | 7 | 8 | 9 | 10 | 11 |

BASAL BODY TEMPERATURES

High

35 F C

Lower Baseline BBT

| | 7 | 8 | 9 | 10 | 11 | 12 | 13 | 14 | 15 | 16 | 17 | 18 | 19 | 20 |

Nasreen notices this start-stop pattern with her fluids and drew this squiggle line to point it out. She decides to follow up with her provider to check in on this.

BODY FLUIDS

CYCLE DAY	1	2	3	4	5	6	7	8	9
Bleeding	●	●	●	○	○	○	○	○	○
Spotting	○	○	●	●	○	○			
Dry	○	○	○	○	○	○			
Creamy	○	○	○	○	○	●	●		○
Slippery	○	○	○	○	○	○	○	●	○

CATEGORIES

CYCLE DAY	1	2	3	4	5	6	7	8	9	10	11	12	13	14	15	16	17	18	19	20
1 Comfort	○	○	○	●	●	●	○	●	●	○										
2 OPK	○	○	○	○	○	○	11	6	7	6	10	11	8	4	13	6	3	○		
3																				
4																				
5																				
6																				

The instructions in Nasreen's OPK said to expect a "surge" at 25. She notices that her highest number is 13. She draws another squiggle here to share this with her provider.

12 13 14 15 16 17 18 19 20 21 22 23 24 25 26 ___ ___ ___ ___ DATE **MAY** MONTH

Drawing a line in the middle (or average) of the entire cycle's BBTs can help point out where significant hormone shifts may have occurred. Many people experience a lower average BBT in the follicular phase and a higher average BBT in the luteal phase. Typically, this looks a cluster of lower temperatures on the left side of your cycle and a cluster of higher temperatures on the right side of your cycle.

6 37 38 39 40 CYCLE DAY

Higher Baseline BBT

36 F C

BASAL BODY TEMPERATURES

Nasreen expected a clearer cluster of low and high BBTs. In fact, she doesn't really see a significant rise in temperature at all. Nasreen also flags this to share with her provider.

Lower Baseline BBT

35 F C

CYCLE DAY	21	22	23	24	25	26	27	28	29	30	31	32	33	34	35	36	37	38	39	40	
	○	○	○	○	○	○	○	○	○	○	○	○	○	○	○	○	○	○	○	○	Bleeding
	○	○	○	○	○	○	○	○	○	○	○	●	●	●	○	○	○	○	○	○	Spotting
	○	○	○	●	○	○	○	○	○	○	○	○	○	○	○	○	○	○	○	○	Dry
	○	○	○	○	●	○	○	○	○	○	○	○	○	○	○	○	○	○	○	○	Creamy
	○	○	○	○	○	○	○	○	○	○	○	○	○	○	○	○	○	○	○	○	Slippery

BODY FLUIDS

CYCLE DAY	21	22	23	24	25	26	27	28	29	30	31	32	33	34	35	36	37	38	39	40		
	○	○	○	○	○	○	○	○	○	○	○	○	○	○	○	○	○	○	○	○	Comfort	1
	○	○	○	○	○	○	○	○	○	○	○	○	○	○	○	○	○	○	○	○	*OPK*	2
	○	○	○	○	○	○	○	○	○	○	○	○	○	○	○	○	○	○	○	○		3
	○	○	○	○	○	○	○	○	○	○	○	○	○	○	○	○	○	○	○	○		4
	○	○	○	○	○	○	○	○	○	○	○	○	○	○	○	○	○	○	○	○		
	○	○	○	○	○	○	○	○	○	○	○	○	○	○	○	○	○	○	○	○		5
	○	○	○	○	○	○	○	○	○	○	○	○	○	○	○	○	○	○	○	○		
	○	○	○	○	○	○	○	○	○	○	○	○	○	○	○	○	○	○	○	○		6

CATEGORIES

CYCLE

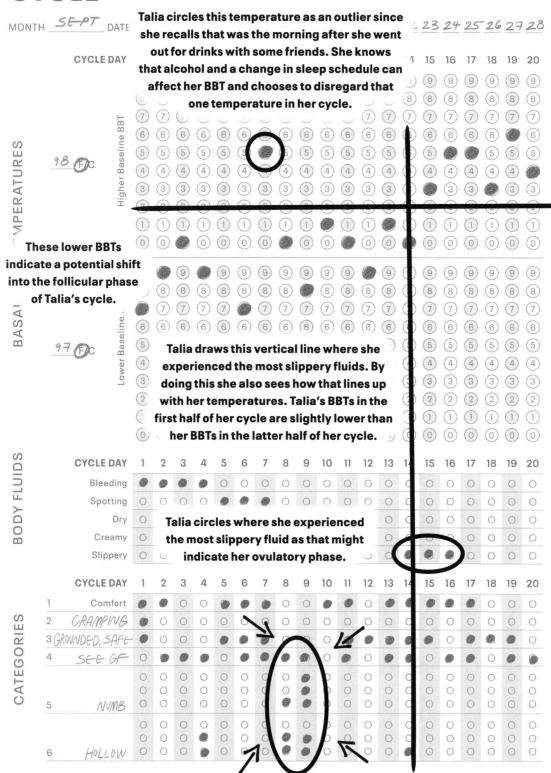

MONTH _SEPT_ DATE

CYCLE DAY

Talia circles this temperature as an outlier since she recalls that was the morning after she went out for drinks with some friends. She knows that alcohol and a change in sleep schedule can affect her BBT and chooses to disregard that one temperature in her cycle.

23 24 25 26 27 28

14 15 16 17 18 19 20

TEMPERATURES

BASAL

Higher Baseline BBT

98 F/C

These lower BBTs indicate a potential shift into the follicular phase of Talia's cycle.

Lower Baseline

97 F/C

Talia draws this vertical line where she experienced the most slippery fluids. By doing this she also sees how that lines up with her temperatures. Talia's BBTs in the first half of her cycle are slightly lower than her BBTs in the latter half of her cycle.

BODY FLUIDS

CYCLE DAY	1	2	3	4	5	6	7	8	9	10	11	12	13	14	15	16	17	18	19	20
Bleeding	●	●	●	○	○	○	○	○	○	○	○	○	○	○	○	○	○	○	○	○
Spotting	○	○	○	○	●	●	●	○	○	○	○	○	○	○	○	○	○	○	○	○
Dry	○													○	○	○	○	○	○	○
Creamy	○													○	○	○	○	○	○	○
Slippery	○	○							○	○	●	●	○	○	○	○	○	○	○	○

Talia circles where she experienced the most slippery fluid as that might indicate her ovulatory phase.

CATEGORIES

CYCLE DAY	1	2	3	4	5	6	7	8	9	10	11	12	13	14	15	16	17	18	19	20
1 Comfort	●	●	○	○	●	●	●	○	○	●	●	○	●	●	●	●	●	○	○	○
2 CRAMPING	●	○	○	○	○	○	○	○	○	○	○	○	○	○	○	○	○	○	○	○
3 GROUNDED, SAFE	●	○	○	○	○	○	○	○	○	●	●	●	○	●	●	○	●	●	●	○
4 SEE GF	○	●	○	●	●	●	●	●	●	○	○	○	○	○	●	●	○	●	●	●
	○	○	○	○	○	○	○	○	●	○	○	○	○	○	○	○	○	○	○	○
	○	○	○	○	○	○	○	○	●	○	○	○	○	○	○	○	○	○	○	○
5 NUMB	○	○	○	○	○	○	○	●	●	○	○	○	○	○	○	○	○	○	○	○
	○	○	○	●	○	○	○	●	●	○	○	○	○	○	○	○	○	○	○	○
6 HOLLOW	○	○	○	●	○	○	●	●	●	○	○	○	○	○	○	○	○	○	○	○

29 30 1 2 3 4 5 6 7 8 9 __ __ __ __ __ __ __ __ __ __ DATE **OCT** MONTH

BASAL BODY TEMPERATURES

CYCLE DAY: 21 22 23 24 25 26 27 28 29 30 31 32 33 34 35 36 37 38 39 40

Higher Baseline BBT

These higher BBTs indicate a potential shift into the luteal phase of Talia's cycle.

98 F/C

Talia draws this horizontal line through what looks like the middle of all of her BBTs. By comparing the shifts above and below that line, she can start to see where her follicular and luteal phases might be.

Lower Baseline BBT

97 F/C

BODY FLUIDS

CYCLE DAY: 21 22 23 24 25 26 27 28 29 30 31 32 33 34 35 36 37 38 39 40

Bleeding
Spotting
Dry
Creamy
Slippery

CATEGORIES

CYCLE DAY: 21 22 23 24 25 26 27 28 29 30 31 32 33 34 35 36 37 38 39 40

Comfort 1
CRAMPING 2
GROUNDED, SAFE 3
SEE GF 4

NUMB 5

HOLLOW 6

When Talia is scanning her chart to see if there are clusters of filled in bubbles, she notices a pattern. She sees high rates of intensity bubbles for numb and hollow following consecutive days that she saw her girlfriend. Talia circles this as she wants to explore it further. She wonders if she may be able to rule out a hormonal connection to the numb and hollow feelings she's been tracking.

14.

Anatomy

Anatomy is not always universal, nor is it static.

Every person and every body is unique. Some people have only some of the following parts, while others have variations of them. And even within a single person, anatomy can change with age, hormonal shifts, or hormone therapy.

The following is a glossary of some body parts that may be relevant to your cycle. You can see or touch many of these parts on the outside of your body, and we refer to these as external. We refer to anatomy inside your body as internal—parts that you may be able to see and feel through methods described below.

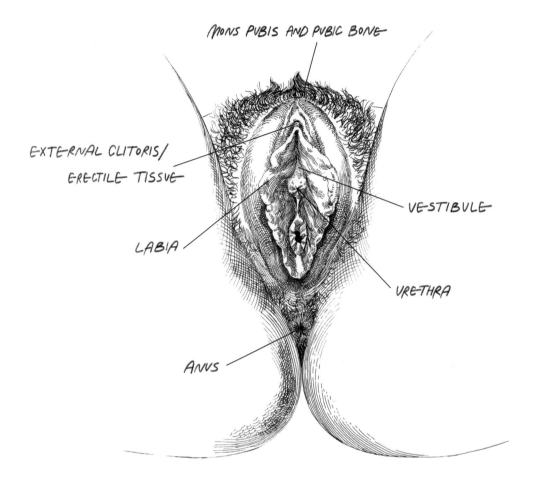

MONS PUBIS AND PUBIC BONE

EXTERNAL CLITORIS/
ERECTILE TISSUE

VESTIBULE

LABIA

URETHRA

ANUS

ANUS The anus is the opening end of the gastrointestinal tube that allows solid waste to exit the body. You can feel and see your anus on the outside of your body. A mirror can help you see this part.

CERVIX The cervix is the lower portion of the uterus. It is tunnel shaped and acts as a pathway between the body of the uterus and the vagina. During the follicular and luteal phases, the cervical opening closes and firms, so it may feel closer to your vaginal opening at these times than during ovulation. During ovulation, the cervix softens, slightly opens, and produces a clear, slippery fluid. You can feel your cervix by inserting a clean finger into the vagina, or you can see your cervix by using a speculum and a mirror.

CLITORIS/EROGENOUS TISSUE
The clitoris is a sexual stimulation organ that can range in size, length, and width, often measuring approximately 9–11 centimeters. The very tip of it is positioned above the urethral and vaginal openings. The body of this organ, however, extends inside your body, beneath the labia. The clitoris includes erectile tissue that can change and swell as it fills with blood. It has over ten thousand nerve endings throughout the organ. The clitoris can be sensitive to many types of touch, pressure, and vibration, allowing for stimulation and pleasure. You can see the tip of your clitoris outside of the body by using a mirror. You feel the external clitoris by using a clean finger to touch the tip of your clitoris and your clitoral hood, both of which are near your vestibule. While you may not be able to see the aspects of the internal clitoris, you can use gentle pressure with this clean finger to explore sensations around your vulva and inside your vagina.

EXTERNAL CLITORIS/ERECTILE TISSUE
The external clitoris is positioned above the urethral opening where the labia meet. It's protected by the clitoral hood, which is a fold of skin that covers it. You can see and touch the external clitoris. You can consider this the head of the clitoris.

INTERNAL CLITORIS/ERECTILE TISSUE
Composing 90 percent of the clitoris, the internal organ includes the body, legs, and bulbs, which all come together in one area by the urethra. Many believe this area to be what is commonly referred to as the G-spot. The internal clitoris extends internally below the labia, around the vaginal wall, and toward the anus. The close proximity of the internal clitoris to the vaginal walls can allow for arousal and sensitivity to vaginal touch. While you can't see the internal clitoris, you might notice the feelings associated with the internal clitoris through touch.

CORPUS LUTEUM The corpus luteum is the structure that the follicle creates after it has released an egg cell. Its function is to produce hormones that plump the uterine lining. Once the corpus luteum has done its job, it dissolves in place. The corpus luteum can be seen via ultrasound imaging. Some people feel a subtle or sharp abdominal ache or twinge connected to different stages of the corpus luteum's lifespan during or around ovulation.

FOLLICLE Follicles are fluid-filled cases inside the ovaries that act as protectors and transporters of egg cells and produce hormones during a cycle. A follicle can be seen using ultrasound imaging. Most people don't have physical sensation related to their follicles.

GREATER VESTIBULAR GLANDS The greater vestibular glands are fluid-secreting organs located near the lower opening of the vagina that regulate moisture and lubrication in the vagina. These glands are internal and typically can't be seen without specialized medical imaging or felt through touch. If these glands become swollen you may be able to feel them through your skin. These are also referred to as Bartholin's glands; however, we prefer *greater vestibular glands*, which describes the anatomy rather than the anatomist who claimed them.

HYMEN The hymen is a thin membrane located at the bottom of the vaginal opening that changes in shape and consistency over a lifetime. Not everyone has a hymen, and its societal association with virginity and sexual activity is inaccurate. As a concept, virginity doesn't accurately represent a person's experience with sexuality and is based solely on the idea of penetrative sex. A person's sexuality is much more expansive and may never include penetration. While the hymen has taken on socially imposed meaning, the function of it in the body is currently unknown. The hymen might be seen with a speculum and a mirror and might be felt by inserting a clean finger into your genital opening.

LABIA   Labia are folds of skin at the vaginal opening. They're part of the vulva and can change in shape and size throughout a lifetime. Their length, thickness, texture, or hair growth vary from person to person. They are protective, keeping contaminants out of the vaginal microbiome, and support nonabrasive vaginal penetration. You can see and touch the labia on the outside of the body.

MONS PUBIS AND PUBIC BONE   The mons pubis is a collection of fatty tissue that sits in front of the pubic bone. It can be seen and touched externally. The pubic bone is the front and center region of your pelvis. It is a junction of your hip bones, which meet with connective cartilage. You can feel the pubic bone just below the surface of your mons pubis by pressing gently.

OOCYTES   Oocytes are immature egg cells that people are born with. Over time the number of oocytes a body has continues to reduce as they are either reabsorbed into the body or released by the body through ovulation. Most people born with oocytes start with over a million. By the time the body reaches puberty, most people have around four hundred thousand oocytes. At the start of menopause that number can reduce to fewer than ten thousand.

OVUM   An ovum (egg cell) is a matured oocyte. It is the singular cell in the body that, if combined with a sperm cell, has the potential to lead to a pregnancy. If we only notice or value ova for this reproductive function, we may miss the opportunity to engage with the cycle even when, or if, we're not interested in procreation. Ova play an imperative role in your body's hormonal function all the time. An egg cell is the biggest cell in the body. While it can be seen with the naked eye, it is best viewed with a microscope. Most people do not have sensations associated with ova.

OVARY   Located at the top of the uterine tubes, the ovaries grow and store egg cells and produce estrogens and progesterone hormones. Ovaries can be seen with ultrasound technology. Most people do not have sensation associated with their ovaries. Some people may have physical feelings around their ovaries with ovulation.

PELVIC FLOOR

The pelvic floor is a muscle system that stretches from the tailbone to the pubic bone, holding up the bladder, uterus, and bowel and providing openings (sphincters) for the urethra, vagina, and anus. Because these muscles support your organs, injuring or straining the pelvic floor can cause significant changes in daily function, including but not limited to feeling pain, incontinence, constipation, and discomfort during sex. Chest binding, pregnancy, and childbirth are just a few of the things that can cause strain on the pelvic floor. The pelvic floor muscle system is internal and can't usually be seen.

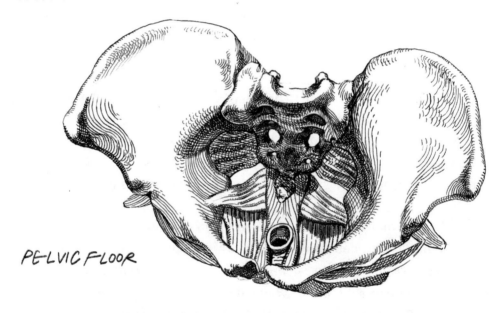

PELVIC FLOOR

PELVIC FLOOR THERAPY

If you're thinking kegels, think bigger. Pelvic floor physical therapists can identify and manage pain or dysfunction associated with the muscle system through exercises, postural changes, and changes to the way you breathe.

EXAMINATION

A pelvic floor specialist can differentiate and examine the pelvic floor muscles through touch. This physical exam typically involves the provider inserting a gloved finger or fingers into the vagina and/or rectum to evaluate the status of your pelvic floor. These professionals can teach you to use your own finger or fingers to feel your pelvic floor yourself.

PERIURETHRAL GLANDS The periurethral glands are fluid-secreting organs located next to the urethra that regulate moisture and lubrication in the urethra. These glands are internal and typically can't be seen or felt. If these glands become swollen, you may be able to feel them through your skin. These are also referred to as Skene's glands; however, we prefer *periurethral glands*, which describes the anatomy rather than the anatomist who claimed them.

URETHRA The urethra is a small hole located above the vaginal opening. It's a tube that allows urine to come from the bladder and out of the body. Some people's urethra can be seen with a mirror, while others' can't. The urethra can be touched and felt with a finger.

UTERUS The uterus is a muscular organ, similar in size and shape to an upside-down pear, located inside the lower abdomen, which builds a lining of blood and tissue during each cycle. The uterus sends that lining out through the vagina during the bleeding phase of each cycle. If a combined sperm and egg cell implants in that uterine lining, it may result in a pregnancy. You can see the uterus through ultrasound imaging. Typically, the uterus is tucked behind the pubic bone. There are a number of circumstances in which the uterus is large enough that you can feel it. Some examples include pregnancy, postpartum, adenomyosis, and fibroids. In these cases, you can feel the uterus above your pubic bone by gently pressing your lower abdomen with your fingertips. A provider may also examine it through external touch, by pressing in the same way with their hands. There may also be an internal sensation associated with the uterus during phases of the menstrual cycle as the uterine muscle actively pushes out lining. Cramping is one of these sensations.

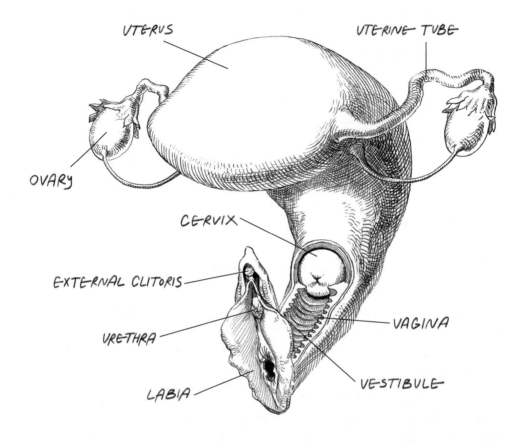

UTERINE LINING Otherwise known as the endometrium, the uterine lining is a layer of blood, tissue, and nutrients that forms along the walls of the uterus. The uterine lining will leave the body at the end of the cycle. The uterine lining can be seen and felt as it exits the body and can be visualized on an ultrasound.

UTERINE TUBES The uterine tubes or salpinges attach to both the ovaries and the uterus. It's not easy to see uterine tubes with ultrasound, so some providers use specialized dye in conjunction with imaging to highlight this area. Most people do not have sensation associated with the uterine tubes.

These are also commonly referred to as Fallopian tubes; however, we prefer *uterine tubes*, which describes the anatomy rather than the anatomist who claimed them.

VAGINA The vagina is a muscular tunnel that begins at the vulva and leads up to your cervix, connecting the external body parts with the internal. It's an incredibly elastic system that can change in shape and size, depending on hormonal shifts, stimulation, or birth. The vagina has a sophisticated self-cleaning system produced through varying body fluids and boasts its own microbiome. You can feel and touch the vagina internally by inserting a clean finger and/or see it by using a mirror and speculum.

VESTIBULE The vestibule is the area between the labia and the vagina and urethra. The vestibular skin is unique in that it may be less elastic than vaginal tissue, has extra nerve endings, and has hormonal cell receptors for estrogen, progesterone, and testosterone. You can feel the vestibule with clean fingers and see it with a mirror.

VULVA The parts of your genitals that are on the outside of your body, including the clitoris, labia, urethra, and vaginal opening, are a group referred to as the vulva. The term comes from the Latin word meaning *covering*, but there is quite a bit more going on with the vulva. It has an extraordinary amount of nerve endings. The vulva is supported by the pelvic floor muscles. This area of the body has the ability to hold a great deal of sensations. You can see your vulva by using a mirror and you can feel and touch your vulva externally with clean fingers.

15.

Body Fluids

It is not surprising to us that the people we work with often express squeamishness or embarrassment when we begin discussions around body fluids, lubrication, and discharge. Just consider the lack of actual representation of this natural body process in any media or mainstream conversations. So many of us have internalized shame or have learned to quickly ignore the body fluids that we do notice.

Vaginal discharge and *cervical mucus* can carry inaccurate stigmas related to dirtiness and odor. The sociocultural baggage around these terms often causes many of us to be uncomfortable with the presence of our own body fluids, ignore them, or even pathologize ourselves.

But all bodies produce fluids. They're indispensable parts of our bodies' regulating and self-cleaning systems, and their presence, consistency, and color are major indicators of the hormonal cycles our bodies move through. In your tracking charts, you'll notice that we refer to vaginal discharge, cervical fluids, and menstrual blood as *body fluids*. We reference the texture and visuals to describe the type of fluid present. By normalizing all these types of fluids that our bodies create and push out, we are aiming to combat stigma.

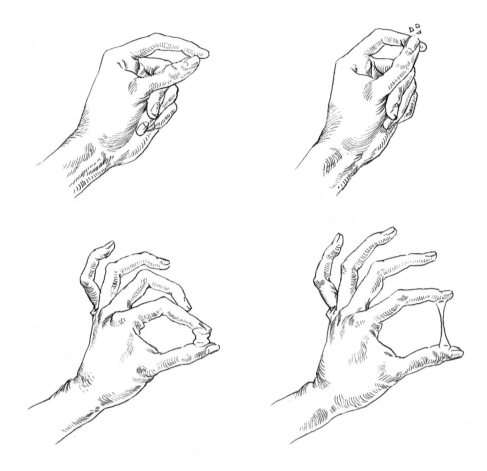

Throughout your cycle, it's completely normal to experience a wide range of body fluids, including menstrual bleeding, discharge, and clear lubrication. The uterus, cervix, and vagina all contribute to different kinds of body fluids at different times, and hormonal shifts can also increase or decrease the amount and type of fluids you might see.

HOW TO CHECK FOR BODY FLUIDS

The most important part of tracking body fluids in and around the vagina is finding a method that feels comfortable and affirming for *you*. Sometimes just noticing body fluids may be a difficult or dysphoric experience. We often hear from our clients how challenging it can be to pay attention to and observe body fluids. If you have experienced trauma, or if others have talked about your body or your identity in ways that don't feel right to you, you may notice that this feels even more uncomfortable, and it might even instigate a disconnect or dissociation. For more about dissociation, see chapter 7, "Dissociation."

If you find that tracking your body fluids feels difficult, be kind to yourself and explore options that feel better, rather than trying to push through something painful. Remember, you are wise and know what feels best for your body. Consider your cues of safety and what feels good.

All ways of monitoring body fluid are equally valid. There's no hierarchy of methods.

Exploring body fluids by inserting a clean finger inside your body may not feel like the safest, most comfortable option—and contrary to popular belief, that's absolutely fine. Although many methods of body fluid observation use an insertion-based approach, there are actually many other meaningful ways to take inventory of fluid changes and shifts.

Make sure to look at the inside of your underwear or clothing at least once a day. What do you see? When observing the wet or dried body fluids, take note of any changes you see in terms of color, density, odor, or amount.

Feel for body fluids when using toilet paper, walking around, or moving throughout your day. When you go to the bathroom, wipe with toilet paper before and after you go. Notice how your body fluids feel when wiping. Does it feel dry? Does the toilet paper slide with the presence of slippery fluid? When you are walking and moving through your day, notice how these fluids feel in your vagina (such as feeling wet or dry). Take note of changes in density, viscosity, or texture.

If insertion is your preferred method of observation, notice body fluids after inserting and removing a clean finger into your vaginal opening to the depth of your comfort. How does the fluid look and feel?

Body Fluid Variations

BLEEDING

To start the follicular phase, the uterine lining detaches from the uterine wall. As it comes off the wall, it produces fluids that might look similar to small blood clots or bleeding from a wound. These fluids are composed of endometrial tissue and blood. This means there is often a wide range of colors, textures, and qualities to this body fluid phase. From person to person, some variation in amount, color (ranging from bright red, brown, dark and rich purpley red, to light pink), or density is completely common.

SPOTTING

Some people experience a smaller amount of blood before, after, or outside the true bleeding phase of the cycle. This typically looks like a little bit of bright red or brown blood on toilet paper when a person wipes, or a spot of blood on their menstrual pad or underwear. We consider this a transitional body fluid, and it's helpful to differentiate it from a fuller flow of bleeding.

DRY

Throughout your cycle, you may find days where your tissues feel drier than they do on other days. This is especially common after bleeding and after ovulation, when the body has finished flushing fluids out of the vagina.

CREAMY

As the body nears the ovulation phase and LH peaks, it's common for body fluids to change to a creamier, more opaque consistency similar to lotion. Throughout the cycle, the vagina continues to act as a self-cleaning system and pushes out unnecessary bacteria and old cells through a creamy fluid.

SLIPPERY

The cervix produces clear and slippery-feeling body fluid before and during ovulation as a way of helping the egg cell move through the uterine tubes. Some people describe this type of fluid as having a lubricating, egg-white-like consistency. If sperm is present in the vagina, this fluid acts as a cleanser. Clean sperm cells enter the uterus by following the trail of body fluid to potentially meet an egg cell. Because this clear body fluid marks ovulation, it holds significance for those focusing on fertility, trying to conceive, or trying to avoid pregnancy. This emphasis on fertility has left a lot of other useful tracking implications around this body fluid out of the dialogue. Clear, slippery fluid and ovulation may also coincide with emotional and physical experiences, such as shifts in arousal, mood, energy, or how it feels to be in the body.

If you notice a color variation or odor that's different from how your fluids normally look or smell, you can use the information you track here to talk with a provider about any imbalances that may be happening in your body. Similarly, if a partner or partners see, smell, or taste anything unusual for you, that can be useful information for you to look into.

16.

Basal Body Temperature (BBT)

Temperature is the part of tracking that nobody wants to do, as it can feel like an annoying chore. That the *basal* part of it is an even bigger ask than taking a straight daily temp is a real barrier. But this is also an extremely helpful bit of data to gather, so we've tried to make it as simple and easy as possible. We love charts that include this data set. BBTs help create a full picture of your body's cycles. It's not so bad!

Basal body temperature (BBT) describes your temperature when you're at a resting state. This temperature data set gives you a baseline for identifying hormonal fluctuations.

The temperature shift your body undergoes throughout your cycle can be subtle, but you may notice a slight increase in BBT of about 0.3°C or 0.5°F, right after ovulation and during the luteal phase. This is largely due to estrogen decreasing and progesterone increasing during these phases, which is why tracking your temperature as a biomarker is a great way to learn more about hormonal peaks and valleys throughout your cycle.

Typically, you can use BBT to confirm when ovulation has occurred, though it's a common misconception that you can *predict* ovulation by tracking temperatures. Temperatures vary from day to day, and the temperature shift that's brought on by hormonal changes is slight, so trying to predict cycle patterns based on daily BBT changes doesn't really work.

We recommend only using BBT as retrospective data alongside other sensation tracking. This means you can look back at past cycles and use BBT shifts to mark suspected times of ovulation, but you can't effectively predict ovulation by taking your temperature in a cycle and using a day-to-day shift. It's just too subtle.

TAKING YOUR BBT

Finding your BBT is about keeping it simple and checking your temperature with no environmental interference. All you'll need is a thermometer that reads in 0.1° increments and doesn't round the decimal number to the nearest whole. To achieve the most accurate results, take your temperature when you're at a full resting state, which is typically after you've been sleeping or lying still for approximately four hours.

Ideally, you'll want to take your temperature at the same time every day—before sitting up in bed, talking, or drinking water in the morning—to ensure that you track consistent numbers over time. Even these seemingly inconsequential actions increase your blood circulation and can raise your temperature. Remember, BBT shifts in a cycle are subtle.

Keeping *The Cycle Book* and your thermometer near where you rest can make tracking BBT as simple as possible.

Georgia

Georgia is a BBT pro—she used tracking to help best time her efforts to conceive her three children, and she is now using tracking to help her figure out her cycle. She recently started menstruating again after the birth and subsequent nursing of her third child. Even though there is often a small person in her bed when she wakes up, she has practiced reaching for her thermometer, which she keeps right on her nightstand, when she opens her eyes.

She quickly takes a temp before she is summoned to pick up a fallen stuffed animal or called to help another small child in the bathroom. Her copy of The Cycle Book *is on her nightstand with a pen inside, although she has been known to use a marker or a crayon if she finds one of those lying around instead. She swiftly fills in her temp bubble, puts* The Cycle Book *back down, and gets out of bed. Georgia's BBT data has allowed her to get really specific in understanding her hormonal shifts, aiding her throughout her fertility experiences as well as in managing and supporting her focus and attention.*

Georgia usually fills out the rest of her chart right before bed. Because bedtimes can often be hectic, she keeps The Cycle Book *close by and fills in her daily bubbles when she gets into bed at night. Georgia has been using the* comfort *tracking category to capture the feeling of returning to herself, albeit in a new way, after weaning. There is something that feels peaceful and relieving for Georgia about finding a new rhythm and relationship to herself.*

Once you've logged a few cycles' worth of BBT data, look at the patterns across your charts and take note of anything that might have impacted your results, including illness, sleep disturbances, stress, or alcohol use. Observing changes over time can be wildly informative and tell you key things about your hormonal patterns.

Tracking your BBT every day is a big ask, so people often experiment with BBT by tracking for two to three cycles to see what they learn about their bodies. You don't have to log your BBT forever to get key information about your hormones. Tracking even a few cycles can be helpful. If you're unable to track a temperature for a certain amount of time, don't worry. Continuing BBT tracking, even with a few gaps, will still provide valuable information.

17.

Birth Control

Generally, there are some basic methods of birth control based on mechanical function—preventing sperm cells from reaching egg cells, preventing sperm from being produced, preventing egg cells from being produced, keeping sperm and egg cells out of the uterus entirely, and stopping a pregnancy from developing in the uterus.

Even though we call these methods *birth control*, many people use these methods to manage difficult hormonal symptoms totally unrelated to their feelings about pregnancy. No matter the reason you are using any of these methods, tracking is helpful.

Mei

Mei finishes her first cycle of tracking her skin, her moods, and her arousal and fantasies after discontinuing her hormonal birth control pill. Even though one of her motivations for this whole endeavor was understanding her moods, she finds herself not even vaguely curious about these fluctuations. Mei has noticed that her skin has started to feel different during her first cycle of tracking, and she starts recalling tough moments in high school when she struggled with her skin. She finds herself preoccupied by some of these memories and realizes that for right now, she feels most motivated to understand how her hormones might impact her skin.

Mei uses the comfort tracking category to reflect days in which she feels a sense of calm within herself that tells her she doesn't really need to go overboard worrying about the impacts of hormones on her body and life. She came into tracking with a lot of things she was worried she would have to "solve," and she has realized that her fears were causing her to feel further away from herself. She tracks comfort to remind herself that she does actually know herself well and can relax while tracking.

As Mei supports herself in determining what her tracking priorities are, she decides to find a dermatologist to help her explore what she's experienced with her skin. She adjusts her tracking accordingly. She sets up consultation appointments with various dermatological providers and continues tracking to have robust information to take with her to these meetings.

Different forms of contraceptives have varying rates of efficacy. People may use more than one birth control method at the same time. Since the way you use and implement each form of contraception impacts its usefulness, try considering what might work best for you, and then explore how using it would look in practice.

If you are using any method of birth control or transitioning on or off one of these methods, *The Cycle Book* can act as your data storage.

KEEPING SPERM CELLS AWAY FROM EGG CELLS

Fertility Awareness Method (FAM)

Fertility awareness methods (FAMs) are forms of contraception that often involve tracking basal body temperature, body fluids, and calendar days to identify the window in which a pregnancy is most likely to occur if sperm is present. The goal of using FAMs to avoid pregnancy is to identify when ovulation will occur and avoid having semen enter the vagina during a variable fertile window before and during ovulation. Semen can survive inside the vagina for up to five days, so this is a nuanced form of birth control that requires careful attention. Depending on which method of FAM a person uses (there are quite a few to choose from), there are set criteria for engaging with biomarkers to designate the window of fertility during each cycle.

TRACKING RECOMMENDATIONS:

When using a chosen FAM method, be sure to stay consistent with the identified criteria for assessing fertile windows.

1. Track beyond biomarkers, including additional physical and emotional sensations, particularly around ovulation. This form of birth control is precise and requires awareness of quite a lot of your own bodily cues to help identify your fertile window in real time. FAMs also require ongoing diligence in tracking because your fertile window, like your cycle, is not the same every time.

2. We find that it takes clients awhile—multiple cycles or longer—to gather enough information to be able to reliably use their chosen FAM. We recommend trying FAMs in combination with other birth control methods like withdrawal, barriers (condoms, diaphragms, cervical caps, sponges, etc.), and then tracking when you use each of those supportive methods.

Withdrawal

Also known as the pull-out method, this form of birth control refers to the practice of withdrawing or pulling a penis out of a vagina, prior to ejaculation. When ejaculation happens away from the vagina and external vulva, semen is unable to enter the body. Withdrawal is often used in conjunction with other contraceptive methods.

TRACKING RECOMMENDATIONS:

The efficacy of this method is dependent on the person in control of semen.

1. If you're using this as a method of contraception, we recommend also tracking the times you had penetrative sex during your cycle.

2. If you are planning repeated sessions of penetrative sex, efficacy of this method may be impacted by the presence of residual semen in the penis. One way to attempt to minimize this risk is for the person with the penis to urinate after ejaculating.

Barrier Method

Barrier methods of birth control include condoms, diaphragms, cervical caps, and sponges—all of which stop semen in its tracks so that sperm can't enter the cervix. Many of these barrier forms also use contraceptive gels or spermicides to increase their effectiveness.

TRACKING RECOMMENDATIONS:

Create a category (or categories) related to vaginal sensations after barrier use and track what you notice. Depending on what materials are used in these barrier methods, many people find that some products cause more or less vaginal irritation.

1. Track the presence of vulval or vaginal irritation throughout the cycle as well as any moments of discomfort or pain with penetration.

Contraceptive Gel and Spermicide

Contraceptive gels and spermicides are chemicals placed directly in the vagina that inhibit pregnancy from occurring by both physically blocking sperm and disrupting their ability to move. These chemicals are often used with barrier methods.

TRACKING RECOMMENDATIONS:

Try tracking any observed changes in your body fluids when using contraceptive gel or spermicide. Many people have varying reactions to the ingredients in these products. By tracking these sensations, you can find products that support your body, your pH, and your vaginal microbiome.

1. Track body fluid changes in amount, color, and consistency, as well as whether you experience any vaginal burning or itching throughout the cycle.

Vasectomy

A vasectomy is a sometimes reversible surgical procedure to block the pathway of sperm exiting a body along with semen.

TRACKING RECOMMENDATIONS:

Vasectomies are not instantly effective and require thoughtful medical follow-up and examination with a surgical team to confirm the success of the operation.

1. If you are having penetrative sex with someone who has had a vasectomy, for birth control purposes, it is crucial to be aware of the amount of time since the procedure, whether their semen was analyzed to confirm that no sperm are present, and whether the follow-up examination was completed.

KEEPING SPERM CELLS FROM BEING PRODUCED

Hormonal Birth Control

There are multiple clinical trials for hormonal birth control to suppress sperm production. These trials have not become mainstream, at least in part due to test subjects' reported frustration with hormonal birth control side effects.

KEEPING EGG CELLS FROM BEING PRODUCED

Hormonal Birth Control

The two types of hormonal birth control that keep eggs from being produced—combined estrogens and progesterone, and progesterone only—work by suppressing ovulation and altering body fluids to be less conducive to semen and pregnancy.

There are many ways to introduce hormonal birth control to the body, including through an implant, an intrauterine device (IUD), an injection, a patch, a ring, or an oral pill. Taking time to consider how to use each form will help you determine which best resonates with you and your lifestyle.

TRACKING RECOMMENDATIONS:

Hormonal birth control introduces new hormones into your body and keeps your body from producing its own. Hormonal shifts of any kind can impact every part of one's mind and body, so tracking while on, transitioning onto, transitioning off, or changing to another form of hormonal birth control can help you understand and manage side effects. (For more information about hormones, see chapter 10, "Hormones.")

1. Assess what type of hormonal birth control might be best for you. When evaluating which type of hormonal birth control you might choose, consider monitoring sensations like mood, sexual arousal, discomfort, bleeding, pain, and chest tenderness. Your personal health history is an important part of the risk assessment around hormonal birth control selection.

2. Use your tracking data to talk to your provider. As you track effects of your hormonal birth control, you may notice a flat-looking chart with few waves of variation. This visual may be showing you the effects of your hormonal birth control.

3. If you want to change your hormonal birth control method, track both wanted and unwanted effects. A simple way to start this inquiry is by tracking one wanted and one unwanted category for three full cycles.

Emergency Contraception

Taking an emergency contraceptive pill (also known as the morning-after pill), such as Plan B or ella, is a form of birth control. It may be taken up to five days after genital exposure to semen, but is more effective if taken within three days. These pills work by using progesterone hormones to stop ovulation from occurring. IUDs are intrauterine devices that are inserted through the cervix into the uterus to stop sperm from reaching an egg. An IUD can be placed within five days of exposure, and once it has been inserted, it can remain in place as a form of long-term birth control.

TRACKING RECOMMENDATIONS:

After using an emergency contraceptive, it's common for people to report changes in their cycles.

1. Tracking your body fluids as well as possible side effects like nausea, fatigue, chest tenderness, bleeding, or pain can help you navigate this transition.

KEEPING SPERM AND EGG CELLS OUT OF THE UTERUS

Intrauterine Device (IUD)

An IUD is a small device that is placed inside the uterus for longer-term birth control. It is reversible upon removal. It is theorized that the materials IUDs are made of (copper, metal, or plastic) create inflamed environments less suitable for sperm and pregnancy. IUDs may also include the hormone progesterone.

TRACKING RECOMMENDATIONS:

It may take some time after IUD insertion or removal for your body to feel like it usually does.

1. Tracking abdominal discomfort, bleeding, spotting, digestive and any other bodily changes with an IUD placement or removal provides you with a set of useful information to help manage possible symptoms and make choices.

Salpingectomy or Tubal Ligation

Tubal ligation is a surgical procedure that closes off the uterine tubes, also known as the salpinges. Salpingectomy is a surgical procedure that removes a portion of the uterine tubes. With both procedures the pathway for egg cells to enter the uterus is blocked off.

TRACKING RECOMMENDATIONS:

Healing from surgery can be different for everyone.

1. Tracking any physical discomforts, digestion changes, bleeding, and other body fluids can help gauge your body's level of healing.

2. Over time, tracking physical sensation changes around penetration or sexuality may also provide insight to possible effects on your system.

STOPPING A PREGNANCY

Abortion

There are two main types of abortion procedures: a medication abortion, where you take pills to end and expel a pregnancy from the uterus, or an in-clinic procedure, where a provider removes a pregnancy from the uterus. Abortion is not only a form of birth control but also a lifesaving intervention for people experiencing early pregnancy loss and miscarriage.

A medication abortion typically involves misoprostol, a medication that creates uterine contractions to empty the uterus, and mifepristone, a medication sometimes used alongside misoprostol that blocks progesterone production to stop a pregnancy from growing.

While there are variations of in-clinic abortion procedures, they generally involve using suction to stop a pregnancy by removing the pregnancy from the uterus.

TRACKING RECOMMENDATIONS:

The ways people emotionally and physically experience abortion vary.

1. Tracking possible symptoms like bleeding, cramping, and pain during and after an abortion can help confirm the success of a procedure, rule out infection and complications, and identify the need for possible supplemental supports.

2. Try tracking your body fluids to better understand the time of transition as you return to your menstrual cycle.

18.

Fertility Choices

"The whole story of a birth begins with that decision to say *yes*, and the roller coaster that loop-de-loops you to the delivery table or at-home birthing pool or what have you—there is so much in it. All of life, every hope and fear, joy and sadness, the understanding of yourself as a mammal, an embodied animal, is in that story." In her memoir detailing her journey with infertility, Michelle Tea taps into the raw unknowns of fertility and our feelings about our own.

No matter your access point, fertility often ends up being intimately connected to identity. While for some people it feels straightforward and clear, we often hear our clients coping with societal expectations of parenthood combined with personal wishes and hopes for what life is going to look like. This can create a swirl of emotions, making many choices about reproduction feel gut-wrenching, a feeling running in the background at all times. The immense pressure we feel to *know*, put on us by the outside world and ourselves, can be crushing at times.

In *The Mother of All Questions*, Rebecca Solnit describes being interrogated by an interviewer about why she didn't have children: "Just because the question can be answered doesn't mean that anyone is obliged to answer it, or that it ought to be asked. The interviewer's question to me was indecent, because it presumed that women should have children, and that a woman's reproductive activities were naturally public business. More fundamentally, the question assumed that there was only one proper way for a woman to live."

Being as lucky as we are to do the work we do, we get to be up close as our clients approach their own choices around their fertility. This includes the daily internal dialogue that is sometimes quiet, sometimes loud, or sometimes as simple as taking a daily birth control pill. It also includes the moment when they ask themselves if they do or don't want children. Or how they feel when they learn that their partner definitely does or does not. Or when they decide to freeze their eggs. Some explore and use donor eggs or surrogacy to build their family, and some donate their eggs or decide to be a surrogate carrier themselves. We see people contend with the sacrifices involved with parenthood, as well as the pain from their own experiences during childhood. We see people work hard to manage their fears about fertility based on myths consumed about hormonal contraceptives, pregnancy loss, and abortion.

Although clarifying your desire to give birth or not may be as clear as a *yes* or a *no*, many people struggle with the complexities of where these urges originate. Sometimes there is a process of acceptance that leads to a choice that feels less active, and that less-active state can feel good. "Time passing will help make my decision for me." It may be a sense of peace in the not-knowing. Ambivalence is familiar. We see this fertility dissonance regularly. If any of this resonates with you, you are not alone.

Solnit also speaks about an experience more common than is represented in our mainstream dialogue: "I'm not dogmatic about not having kids. I might have had them under other circumstances and been fine—as I am now."

The choices people make about fertility are often the reason they come to cycle tracking. When you know clearly that you are, *yes*, interested in pregnancy, tracking is an amazing tool to begin navigating that path and learning how and when that process best begins within your own body.

When you're unsure and sitting in the *maybe* camp, tracking is invaluable.

When you know that you are squarely in the *no*, tracking is indispensable.

In these scenarios, having a repository of your own cycle data can bolster your confidence in your own body and the choices you are making when you are being asked to claim *yes* or *no* when it comes to your fertility.

DECIPHERING AN INFERTILITY DIAGNOSIS

An estimated one in eight people are diagnosed with infertility. Infertility is a diagnosis, not a state of being.

When your body is not doing something that you want it to, you might feel like you are looking at your body like a broken machine that requires constant tinkering to fix.

This process can become all-consuming. When tracking the body with intense precision, noticing each and every sensation and trying to understand how they relate to chances of conception, each day of waiting can feel like an eternity, with success and failure defined entirely by conception. We see clients who, when they feel like they have no control, become overly strict with themselves, exacting and sometimes punishing, as a way of coping with the unknown timeline ahead of them.

We can't change the fact that this will be hard, but we can change the ways we take care of ourselves during this time. Removing stress is not really an option when negotiating infertility is inherently stressful, even though the pressure to create a stress-free environment when trying to conceive is huge. Understanding commonly recommended parts of the process, naming the testing and treatment options that often get overlooked, and finding ways to include kind self-regard, celebrations for your efforts, and care for yourself when dealing with something so hard can really help.

INFERTILITY SCREENING CRITERIA

Infertility screening criteria used by the medical and insurance systems reference an amount of time passed with an assumed meeting of an egg and sperm cell. (25 years old to 34 years old + 12 months of unprotected penetrative sex or using therapeutic donor insemination + no pregnancies = infertility diagnosis; 35 years old to 39 years old + 6 months of unprotected penetrative sex or using therapeutic donor insemination = infertility diagnosis.) Although these guidelines use an age-based timeframe, it's important to remember that fertility doesn't just turn on and off like a light switch at certain ages but is a broader conversation that involves many considerations. While age is certainly imperative, what this looks like is different for every person.

These infertility criteria also assume that the timing of penetrative sex or insemination has allowed for an egg and sperm cell to meet. Without a full exploration of a person's experience with identifying their ovulation signals, obstacles with timing may be missed in the assessment.

FERTILITY TESTING AND HOW YOUR TRACKING DATA CAN HELP

You'd be shocked how often we encounter *timing* as the culprit to not conceiving. This is understandable given that our pregnancy-prevention-focused sex education doesn't spend a lot of time telling us how to listen to our bodies and identify fertile windows. The apps that so many of our clients have used are highly inaccurate at identifying ovulation and fertile windows. We see our clients startled by how small the fertile window seems because public health initiatives have prioritized pregnancy avoidance instead of teaching us about our bodies.

Recording when you have been trying to conceive on your tracking chart is extraordinarily useful in understanding your efforts. By *trying to conceive*, we mean your attempt to facilitate the meeting of a sperm and egg cell. This may be penetrative sex or a variety of insemination methods. Even when seeing a health provider, we find that timing isn't always accurately assessed. Limited time and resources can mean that providers don't often have the opportunity to dig into individualized factors. This is when tracking can become an effective and easy way to understand if timing is or isn't an issue for you.

Challenges with penetrative sex in general can prevent an egg and sperm cell from meeting. For many, penetration involves navigating emotionally or physically tenuous dynamics. Considering the number of variables at play— erections, the way penetration feels, sexual preferences, possible pain, context that may be less than desirable, pressure to perform, the intersection of mental health and penetration—it is easy to see that finding the right timing is not only about correctly identifying when ovulation occurs. If penetrative sex is your primary method of trying to conceive, you may run into these legitimate hurdles. If you aren't able to comfortably have penetrative sex, or if ejaculation during penetrative sex is a challenge, this is a valid experience you may want to share with your provider. Before moving to higher-level and potentially expensive diagnostic testing, we recommend a thorough exploration of timing.

A number of helpful fertility tests are recommended in most clinical settings. These provide useful information on their own but may not capture the full picture of what's happening to your body. This is where your tracking data, combined with test results, can create a more robust vision of what you are working with.

ASSESSMENTS AND TESTING

The access and availability of fertility assessments and testing is expanding every day. Better health and birth outcomes come from connecting with a provider early. A preconception visit often includes a variety of health screenings as well as fertility assessments. These assessments are meant to clarify whether you sit in the fertile or infertile category to guide your providers' recommendations. Remember, these categories are limited.

As access to medical testing continues to expand and the power of preventive healthcare gains recognition, many of these tests are offered to people with no diagnostic criteria of infertility. In this case, these tests are meant to give a general assessment of a person's potential future fertility forecast. These tests can provide useful information; however, they are a snapshot of what's happening in your body at a moment in time and are best used in combination with other methods of understanding your body, including tracking. We see clients who get some of this early testing receive results that end up having little to no impact on their experience of trying to conceive. There are so many unknowns.

Tracking can often provide critical information about how hormones are being used in your body, which is valuable next to these other common clinical assessments.

SOME COMMONLY OFFERED TESTS

Body Fluid Testing

— Fertility hormone panel

A fertility hormone panel is usually collected through bloodwork measuring levels of estrogen, FSH, LH, prolactin, anti-müllerian hormone (also known as AMH, a hormone related to the number of follicles a person has available in the body), and sometimes thyroid levels. This is usually offered on the third day of the bleeding cycle and tells us what level of hormones are present in your bloodstream on that particular day.

— Progesterone levels

Progesterone levels are usually collected through bloodwork but may also be assessed through urine, seven days after confirmed ovulation. If you are able to identify when you ovulate, you may be able to collaborate with your provider to better time this test. This tells us the amount of progesterone in your bloodstream or urine on that day.

Imaging

— Ultrasound

Ultrasound uses a wand and liquid gel to create an image of internal organs. The wand emits sound waves (that we can't hear) that reverberate against the variable density of our insides. Usually having a full bladder is helpful in making images clearer to see. Ultrasound waves don't travel well through air, so when we use gel and look through a full bladder, the image is much clearer than it would be looking through our intestines full of air. Your provider may request that you arrive at the appointment with a full bladder. That feels different for every person, but it might be two to four 8-ounce glasses of water an hour or so before your appointment. The wand is placed on the body with a small amount of gel to capture an image on a nearby screen of the shapes or your internal organs, including your uterus, ovaries, and even the follicles on your ovaries.

Abdominal ultrasounds
These involve placing the wand on your lower abdomen, right above your pubic bone.

Vaginal ultrasounds
These involve placing a wand within the vagina.

— **Sonohysterogram or hysteroscopy**
This procedure involves inserting fluid into the uterus with a thin, strawlike catheter and viewing it with an ultrasound. The liquid allows you to see a more detailed view of the interior structure of the uterus.

— **Hysterosalpingogram (HSG)**
This procedure involves inserting dye into the uterine tubes that can be seen through an X-ray assessment. The uterine tubes are hard to visualize otherwise, so adding this contrast makes them stand out and helps to assess their structure.

TESTS THAT GET FORGOTTEN

— **Semen analysis**
Far too often, partners and donors are overlooked when assessing infertility causes. This test is done by collecting semen at a clinic or in your home and sending it off to a laboratory to verify the amount, structure, and functionality of sperm present.

BARRIERS TO CONCEPTION

— **Structure**
Conditions that impact the shape of internal organs can sometimes also affect fertility. These include conditions that may block the flow of semen, including infections, scar tissue, or an ejaculatory duct obstruction. Conditions that may

make implantation challenging include adenomyosis, endometriosis, fibroids, polyps, injury, and uterine tube differences.

— **Function**

Certain conditions that change how our bodies work, move, and exist can, in turn, affect how our fertility works, too. When our metabolism is functioning differently, as with diabetes and PCOS, or the way blood flows to our reproductive organs is different, as with hypertension, our reproductive system may not function to its highest capacity. Producing sperm that are mature, can swim, and are shaped in a way that can lead to conception may be challenging.

— **Exposure**

All sorts of factors around us can disrupt fertility, including substances like alcohol and opioids, stress, environmental toxins, lack of access to medical care, and nutrient availability.

WHEN IT'S CALLED INFERTILITY BUT IT'S NOT

— **Access**

We see so many of our queer and solo-parenting clients quickly shuffled into higher-intervention and higher-cost infertility treatments and care because of the assumption that this is one of the primary pathways to sperm. There are other ways to connect with sperm, but in our current system, accessing sperm often requires emotional and intellectual labor, time, financial resources, legal representation, and geographic proximity. Although they may not be mentioned at a doctor's visit, there are many at-home and low-intervention options for insemination.

TRACKING RECOMMENDATIONS:

Once you've officially decided to try to conceive, it can be stressful when it doesn't happen right away. If you've been at this for a long time, we know just how painful the process can feel.

1. Rule out timing as a barrier to conception as a first step. Start by tracking one to three cycles; often just one is enough. The goal is to confidently identify your own specific fertile window. Some people have shorter or longer windows, and the windows don't always occur at the same time in your cycle, but you may be able to identify your own hormonal markers that signal upcoming ovulation.

2. Be thoughtful about the ways you are tracking your body—hyperfocus and constant vigilance can create a difficult dynamic within yourself. Broaden the way you are looking at yourself to go beyond a success/failure narrative only defined by conception. If you know that you tend to fixate on your body, have thoughts that feel compulsive, or notice that tracking is starting to feel hard to control, limit your tracking categories and see if it feels possible to reduce the amount of time spent thinking about your body and charting.

3. If penetrative sex is your primary method of trying to conceive, and if penetration comes with its own hurdles or fatigue for you, consider alternate ways for the sperm and egg cells to meet. For example, try an at-home kit for intracervical insemination (ICI) or talk to a provider about other options. In these cases, spotlighting timing in your tracking is extremely valuable.

4. Build in a tracking category of celebration. There are so many steps and conscious efforts involved in this process, far beyond the big asks of trying to conceive. Coping with tremendous unknowns; taking care of our meaningful relationships; finding the space, capacity, and resources to engage with these interventions; juggling the emotional impact—there is so much that goes on during this time. If we don't acknowledge those efforts, it will be hard to run the marathon. If we can't celebrate what we have accomplished, it is easier to lose ourselves.

PREGNANCY LOSS

Early loss or miscarriage happens way more often than people realize, in about a third of pregnancies. This common experience carries complex emotional weight for many people. Reproductive psychologist Jessica Zucker, in her memoir about her own traumatic pregnancy loss, describes the emotional torture of guilt and shame in addition to grief: "Still, research has shown that *more than half* of people who have been through these ordeals feel guilty. More than a quarter feel shame. And indeed, these concepts somehow have been ingrained in the psyches of countless people who've lost their pregnancies—that their bodies were defective, that they failed, that they somehow did something bad, something wrong. Our culture literally adds insult to injury."

TRACKING RECOMMENDATIONS:

When tracking pregnancy loss, there may be a period of healing when your cycle resets and starts with a different rhythm or pace. Tracking a potential change can be helpful as you get to know this new cycle.

1. Consider tracking categories that feel related to the pregnancy loss, like when the loss occurred, days of bleeding, body sensations, safety, and emotions.

ASSISTED REPRODUCTIVE TECHNOLOGIES (ARTS)

People can use cycle-tracking information alongside many assisted reproductive technologies (ARTs), including fertility medications (e.g., Clomid, letrozole, progesterone), intracervical insemination (ICI), intrauterine insemination (IUI), in vitro fertilization (IVF), egg cell and embryo freezing, and the use of donor eggs.

If using ARTs, timing is everything. Whether you are using medications that narrow or define timing or following the rhythm of your cycle, optimal timing is crucial. Getting specific about ovulation signals can be helpful, particularly in recognizing when your LH reaches elevated levels and your BBT rises. For more information about LH, see chapter 10, "Hormones." To brush up on BBT, see chapter 16, "Basal Body Temperature (BBT)."

When medications are involved in ARTs, tracking related sensations and side effects is useful in creating better individualized support for yourself. Often, ARTs are done sequentially, meaning multiple rounds and attempts at pregnancy occur prior to conception. Tracking sensations through a fertility treatment series is also a great way to verify with your provider whether that particular protocol of ARTs continues to be the best option for you.

TRACKING RECOMMENDATIONS:

Using ARTs as a support for fertility goals can come with some emotional challenges. We often see clients struggle with feelings of personal disconnect, loneliness, and the often grueling side effects of the medications used with ARTs. A handful of specific tracking recommendations in this situation can help:

1. Add a category of support that can mitigate or neutralize stress. If it feels challenging to come up with a category option that works for you, we like to start with the idea that moving the body can move stress out. It doesn't have to be exercise and it doesn't have to be excessively time-consuming—think any type of movement like dance, laughter, sweating, and massage.

2. Consider ways to include anyone else involved with your efforts to conceive—this is not all on you. As you work with others, tracking the ways you have dedicated yourself to those relationships and the shared nature of this endeavor can remind you of the strength of your relationships and the amount of care you put into them.

3. Track the side effects of some of the medications used with ART therapies during and after your course of treatment. This could include abdominal pain and discomfort, hot flashes, chest tenderness, headaches, and moods that feel different or less stable to you.

19.

Perimenopause

"Menopause is a life stage. It's not an illness or progressive disease." Heather Corinna, in their menopause manifesto, *What Fresh Hell Is This?*, is the messenger we are looking for. Over and over they share the message that your body isn't broken—you're changing, and you have new needs.

Any time we live through a physical, metabolic, or hormonal shift, our sense of identity redevelops and redefines. This is a big deal. There is something special about perimenopause in particular, because of the vast experiences under your belt when this shift happens.

NEW PHASES

As longitudinal research into hormones slowly increase, some researchers are proposing new, more specific hormonal stages, potentially including a phase of hormonal variability occurring before perimenopause. For some, this may mean that changes in length of cycles and hormonal shifts may begin in their forties, without yet entering perimenopause.

A familiarity with your hormonal cycle, no matter what that cycle looks like, is something a lot of us come to depend on, consciously or not. To have this cycle begin to change, or even stop, may be a bit discombobulating, like a subtle, nagging feeling that something isn't as it should be. This transition to another "new normal" can also require emotional energy and learning your body's rhythms.

In perimenopause, hormone levels are shifting. As always, these hormones are communicating your body's needs. In this case, your body's needs are likely changing, too.

What has worked for a long time may no longer work in the same way. We are talking about ways to take care of yourself emotionally, physically, relationally, and sexually. Across the board, you may notice that the best ways to take care of yourself may be evolving.

Using tracking can help with new pattern recognition to reassure, affirm, and stabilize you as you ride the waves of this new normal. This being another health experience lacking research, attention, and education, the signs of perimenopause are not always well understood. Without a good idea of what the markers of perimenopause are, you may mistake some of the more gradual impacts of perimenopause for something else or dismiss them altogether. For some, perimenopause starts with a bang, abruptly. For others, it is a lengthy, more subtle shift.

Perimenopause is experienced individually, by each person who is living through it. This phase can last a few months or up to twenty years, with official approximations suggesting a range of three to ten years or more. Some people start perimenopause in their thirties, but for many, the process begins in their forties or fifties. We encourage you to use tracking to identify your own timeline.

Aisha

Aisha had felt like she was losing her mind and her job until tracking helped her see that there were patterns to her symptoms. After reviewing a few months of her charts, Aisha started to explore the idea that her variable cycle lengths and her disrupted sleep might be early signs of perimenopause. She had imagined she would notice perimenopause when it seemed her mom did, in her late forties. At forty-two, the thought had not really been on her mind. She also didn't really know what she had been imagining would happen—the stereotypes were there, the comical hot sweats and the absurd anger—but she wasn't sure what to actually expect.

Aisha starts looking around for a provider who feels like the right fit for the type of support she's looking for. She wants to prioritize her sleep, as she feels that stable sleep is a necessary foundation for everything else in her life. Aisha had thought she would feel stressed about perimenopause, but she actually feels relieved to have a framework to understand how to take care of her body and its current needs. She uses the comfort *tracking category to show possible cycle patterns when she feels a sense of trust in her ability to make good choices for her body. Change motivates Aisha, and she wants to properly cultivate her sense of self and understand her new needs.*

The guidelines around menopause have less to do with personal identity than they do with health parameters, as is evidenced by its clinical definition, which states that the moment in which menopause is "official" is exactly 365 days since the last time you had a period. It is unlikely that this blip in time—the second that Day 364 turns into Day 365—will be the lightning-striking, earth-shaking moment in which you receive your proverbial postmenopausal letter in the mail.

After this moment is realized, you are considered postmenopausal, marked by the cessation of your ovaries cyclically producing hormones and egg cells, and you may notice perimenopausal feelings subsiding.

COMMON IMPACTS

It's easy to get the idea that life in and after menopause is going to be little, dreary rituals of desperate maintenance and exacting control over food, exercise, the shape and size of our bodies, our skin, our intimate relationships, our sexuality, our leisure, our moods, robbing us of what pleasure we might have found in these things before . . . We are not supposed to find freedom, liberation, or a whole new world

of badassery through and on the other side of this. What many of
us so often don't know is that even despite so many barriers
and blockades, a great many people do.

—HEATHER CORINNA, *WHAT FRESH HELL IS THIS?*

Just because something is common or normal does not mean it should be accepted or ignored. Using tracking to better understand the changing needs of your body provides a pathway to seeking any support you may want.

With even less public discourse and education around perimenopause than menstruation, our clients have often experienced symptoms of perimenopause without realizing it since nobody has taught us what to expect.

- **Body changes**
  - ‣ Body pain
  - ‣ Changes in body size and shape
  - ‣ Changes in bone mass and density
  - ‣ Difficulty sleeping or night sweats, especially in the early-morning hours
  - ‣ Gastrointestinal discomfort, such as heartburn, acid reflux, bloating, gas, or changes in bowel movements
  - ‣ Genital pain
  - ‣ Hair changes, such as thinning or facial hair increasing
  - ‣ Headaches or migraines
  - ‣ Hot flashes
  - ‣ Skin changes, such as thinning, drying, or losing collagen
  - ‣ Thinning nails
  - ‣ Urinary tract changes

- **Cognitive shifts**
  - ‣ Changes in memory
  - ‣ Shifts in attention and focus

- **Menstrual impacts**
  - ‣ Changes in the time between menstrual cycles, which typically starts with a reduction in days between cycles, then increases as cycles become further apart

- **Mental or emotional adjustments**
  - ‣ Activation or exacerbation of mental health experiences, such as anxiety, depression, or OCD
  - ‣ Changes in how stress impacts the body and mind
  - ‣ Changes in sexual desire or arousal
  - ‣ Changes of expression of trauma response
  - ‣ Mood shifts, including irritability or anger
  - ‣ Adjustment in identity regarding fertility
  - ‣ Contending with societal value of fertility and reproduction

At any age, if you take certain supplemental hormones or hormone blockers, whether for gender affirmation processes or other health benefits like cancer prevention, you may experience perimenopausal symptoms at earlier ages or in different ways. Similarly, if you have undergone a uterectomy (removal of portions of the uterus or the entire uterus, also called hysterectomy) or oophorectomy (removal of one ovary or both ovaries) or a combination of the two, you may experience signs of perimenopause at a different age.

TRACKING RECOMMENDATIONS:

1. No need to take your basal body temperature—instead, track your own perception of temperature. Hot flashes and night sweats can be a replacement for BBT.

2. Find ways to identify how your new hormonal shifts are expressed. Consider tracking some more common signs of evolving hormones like vaginal discomfort (dryness, irritation), arousal, and mood.

3. Identify the top three changes you are noticing and start by tracking these.

20.

Conclusion

Nasreen

After Nasreen finishes charting and explores her anovulatory patterns with her providers, she is presented with multiple pathways toward pregnancy, many of them being ARTs. She digests her treatment options. She has learned so much about herself and her body as she has tracked and quickly comes to a decision she feels excited about. Nasreen decides that the next step for her is stimulating ovulation through medication. She feels empowered and has renewed energy for her treatment plan. She starts to feel like herself again.

Nasreen continues tracking throughout her ART medicated cycles and is encouraged as she recognizes the presence of ovulation biomarkers and sensations in her cycle. She feels connected to her body and more inclined to listen to it and herself.

Ines

Ines feels equipped to manage her endometriosis diagnosis and take care of her ongoing needs as she identifies them. She notices her shame dissipating as she recognizes the significant barriers she has confronted within the medical system in her journey to diagnosis and treatment.

Ramona

Now if Ramona is having trouble making art in the second half of her cycle, rather than beating herself up about it, she attends to other task-based work in her studio, knowing that it's normal to be feeling this way. She has found a new sense of patience for her body, she has changed her relationship to the pressures of productivity, and her depressive symptoms have lessened.

Mei

Throughout her cycle charting, Mei learns so much about her health priorities. She also learns about her fertility and the signs of when she is ovulating and could possibly become pregnant. An unexpected benefit has been a reduction in stress and pressure as she learns to trust her body. Mei has connected to a dermatologist she likes and is making appointments with providers to explore some different birth control options, possibly without hormones.

Sam

The simple act of tracking small moments of body neutrality and their body's cycles creates more feelings of pleasure for Sam. They are pleasantly surprised to feel a self-critical voice loosen up inside. They feel like they have the power to shift how they feel about their body for the first time and bring this practice into their work with a therapist.

Georgia

When Georgia looks at the results of her charting, she is astounded to see that the frustrating moments with focus, attention, and functioning in her family are occurring like clockwork with her regular hormonal shifts. Georgia is able to set up more support systems preemptively and works with her doctor to find individualized ADHD medication dosing that matches her cycle.

Talia

Talia feels a wave of recognition as she understands that feelings of vulnerability with another person can instigate dissociation for her. She feels kindness toward herself and comfort in the fact that she has made meaning of this. She brings this up in her support group and is met with a chorus of acknowledgment.

She notices that she feels less frustrated and more connected. Her overall mood improves and her worry reduces. It is not hormonal and definitely not related to her cycle. But it is related to when she sees her girlfriend. Understanding how her hormones impact her (and don't) continues to support Talia's efforts to make informed choices for her own care.

Aisha

Aisha's awareness of her new perimenopausal cycle cadence has given her permission to go easy on herself, understand that the feeling of anxiety won't last forever, and be thoughtful around her own expectations. She has stopped the extra check-ins with her boss because she feels strong in the knowledge that she can soothe herself.

In a sea of misinformation, a confusing array of competing treatment options, an overburdened healthcare system, troubling systemic bias, and endless predatory health influencers, the information you've gathered here is *yours* and it's *real*.

Throughout this book, you have created a way to combat this chaos. You've come up with your own unique method of tuning in to your body, listening to yourself, and finding safety and comfort within your being. You have observed and recorded amazing and important data about yourself. You have prioritized your own version of pleasure.

The stories and information we've shared are based on our personal lived experiences and time in practice with clients. Our hope is that by sharing what we have seen over the years, we are able to save you some time when taking care of your own health and well-being. Ultimately, we hope this book has affirmed your trust in yourself.

You are the true expert in you-ness. Nobody gets to take that away from you. In the ongoing fight to have agency over our own bodies, we encourage you to trust yourself, stay critical, and don't settle.

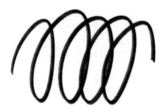

HEALTH APPOINTMENT PREVIEW

Get ready for your next health appointment by organizing your thoughts and goals around your upcoming visit.

GOALS

Goal of my appointment:

_____

_____

Questions I'd like answered:

_____

_____

Symptoms I want to address:

_____

BACKGROUND

These symptoms affect my life in the following ways:

_____

_____

The parts of my life that are impacted include:

○ Mental Health   ○ Physical Body   ○ Fertility   ○ Chronic Condition

○ Pain   ○ Sexuality   ○ Cognition   ○ _____

How my symptoms show up in my cycle:

_____

_____

When my symptoms show up in my cycle:

○ Bleeding Phase   ○ Follicular Phase   ○ Ovulatory Phase   ○ Luteal Phase

Things I've already tried:

_____

_____

MY INSIGHTS

My theory about what is happening in my body:

_____

_____

I'd like to walk away from my appointment with:

○ Prescription　　○ Referral　　○ Diagnosis　　○ Recommendations　　○ Treatment/Management Plan

○ Investigative Testing Plan　　○ Reassurance　　○ Validation　　○ _____

APPOINTMENT REVIEW

Recap and identify what comes next. This may be filled out during or after visit.

What might be causing my current concern?

_____

How might my concern affect the rest of my body?

_____

What are the available treatments for my concern?

_____

Do these treatments have side effects?

_____

What will happen if I do nothing?

_____

Are there other types of providers who specialize in treating these symptoms?

_____

Did this appointment address my needs?　　　　　　　　○ Yes ○ No ○ I'm not sure

Did this provider feel like the right fit for me?　　　　　○ Yes ○ No ○ I'm not sure

NEXT STEPS

What's next for me? My next steps are:

_____

_____

Acknowledgments

Thank you to our clients. This book would not exist without them. Doing this work with you is our greatest privilege.

To our agent, Lindsay Edgecombe. Thank you for being our fearless leader and for your generosity in shaping this project. We had a vision, you turned it into a book. To Nina Shield, Hannah Steigmeyer, and the team at TarcherPerigee, our deepest gratitude for believing in this project and in us.

To those who lent their genius and enthusiasm in the earliest iterations of this project, John Wise, Joel Rubin, Ash Holland, and Anja Slibar, without the foundation you created we wouldn't be here. To Kyle Vereyken, everyone's muse, you know we couldn't have done any of this without you.

To the incredible artists we are also so lucky to be able to call friends, Maxine McCrann and Miles Yoshida, thank you so much for sharing your unbelievable talents with our book.

To Judie, thank you for your medical review from the start. To Luca Harris, FNP, MSN, and Brett Powers, MD, thank you for your medical expertise, guidance, and encouragement.

To Bruce, Morgan's father, thank you for holding our hand through the publishing process and answering every urgent literary call. To Sierra Holland, CPM, PhD, thank you for your meticulous research.

This book is a culmination of many people and their efforts. Thank you to everyone.

Thank you, first, to Morgan, for being in this with me for years. Seeing your face every week has been the biggest gift. This project is a result of your brilliance.

Thank you to my colleagues, supervisors, and doctors throughout the years, who offered such generous and kind support and provided wisdom that entirely shaped this project. Your openhearted, compassionate care continues to inspire me daily. I've learned so much from just being around you all. My heartfelt thanks to Joanna, Mary, Nelly, and Dr. Abby.

To my whole extended family, I couldn't be luckier to have such amazing people in my corner. Thank you to my wonderful brothers for being with me through it all. A huge thank-you to Trina and Jessica—my friends and my family. Rhianna, thank you for your input from the start. Thank you to Ann, Peter, and Suzee. Thank you to the many friends who have navigated the world with me and inspired me through your strength—a special thanks to Haley, Fleur, Shannon, Manuela, Sophie, and the listserv. My deepest gratitude to Ma'any for your invaluable feedback throughout all stages of this project and for so beautifully nurturing the two little people most important to me.

To my parents, who have taught me how to stand up for what matters without giving up, my endless gratitude for always pushing me and showing me how to do hard things. To my beloved daughters, you are both a revelation. I adore you. And to Ariel— the ultimate icon, momager, and shining star. You are the brightest light in my life, thank you.

LAURA

Thank you to the many friends and colleagues who supported this project over the years. To Janette, thank you for midwifing me into being a midwife and modeling the truest form of client-centered care. To the entire Soft Corner Midwifery team, thank you for fueling me through this project amid busy clinic days, sleepless nights, and quite a few new baby birthdays. I'm honored to work alongside such exceptional practitioners and people. To my therapist, Lauren, thank you for so many things, and particularly your expert consult regarding this book. To my darling Jess, thank you for being my friend and sharing the passion of this work.

Enormous gratitude to my family for their tireless encouragement. To my father, Bruce, thank you for persistently believing in me. Your patience and insight as a parent, professional mentor, and friend have meant everything. Thank you for showing me that teaching is sharing and that we should never stop doing it or striving for more connection in the world. To my mother, Cynthia, thank you for your relentless love. Thank you for teaching me to fight against injustice and never give up. Thank you for showing me how to love unconditionally, work hard, and make creativity flourish. To my brother, Grey, thank you always for your love, support, and being you.

To my biggest champion, Joshua, thank you for having endless confidence in me and offering the steadiest encouragement. Thank you for investing in this project with me and helping it come to fruition. Thank you for being my constant sounding board and exemplifying how to stay critical and live and love radically.

And of course, to Laura, thank you for daring to do this with me. Great idea. XOXO.

MORGAN

Recommended Readings

Blair, Gabrielle. *Ejaculate Responsibly: A Whole New Way to Think about Abortion*. New York: Workman, 2022.

Brotto, Lori A. *Better Sex through Mindfulness: How Women Can Cultivate Desire*. Vancouver, BC: Greystone Books, 2018.

brown, adrienne maree. *Pleasure Activism: The Politics of Feeling Good*. Edinburgh: AK Press, 2019.

Brown, Sherronda J., Hess Love, and Grace B. Freedom, *Refusing Compulsory Sexuality: A Black Asexual Lens on Our Sex-Obsessed Culture*. Berkeley, CA: North Atlantic Books, 2022.

Chen, Angela. *Ace: What Asexuality Reveals about Desire, Society, and the Meaning of Sex*. Boston: Beacon Press, 2021.

Clancy, Kate. *Period: The Real Story of Menstruation*. Princeton, NJ: Princeton University Press, 2023.

Coady, Deborah, and Nancy Fish. *Healing Painful Sex: A Woman's Guide to Confronting, Diagnosing, and Treating Sexual Pain*. Berkeley, CA: Seal Press, 2011.

Corinna, Heather. *What Fresh Hell Is This? Perimenopause, Menopause, Other Indignities and You*. London: Piatkus, 2021.

Cleghorn, Elinor. *Unwell Women: Misdiagnosis and Myth in a Man-Made World*. New York: Dutton, 2022.

Criado-Perez, Caroline. *Invisible Women: Data Bias in a World Designed for Men.* New York: Abrams Press, 2021.

Dusenbery, Maya. *Doing Harm: The Truth about How Bad Medicine and Lazy Science Leave Women Dismissed, Misdiagnosed, and Sick.* New York: HarperOne, 2018.

Garbes, Angela. *Like a Mother: A Feminist Journey through the Science and Culture of Pregnancy.* New York: Harper Wave, 2019.

Gunter, Jennifer. *The Menopause Manifesto: Own Your Health with Facts and Feminism.* New York: Kensington, 2021.

Haines, Staci. *Healing Sex: A Mind-Body Approach to Healing Sexual Trauma.* San Francisco: Cleis Press, 2007.

Hendrickson-Jack, Lisa. *The Fifth Vital Sign: Master Your Cycles & Optimize Your Fertility.* Ajax, ON: Fertility Friday, 2019.

Hossain, Anushay. *The Pain Gap: How Sexism and Racism in Healthcare Kill Women.* New York: Simon Element, 2022.

Kali, Kristin Liam. *Queer Conception: The Complete Fertility Guide for Queer and Trans Parents-to-Be.* Seattle: Sasquatch Books, 2022.

Levine, Peter A. *Waking the Tiger: Healing Trauma.* Berkeley, CA: North Atlantic Books, 1997.

Montei, Amanda. *Touched Out: Motherhood, Misogyny, Consent, and Control.* Boston: Beacon Press, 2023.

Nagoski, Emily. *Come as You Are: Revised and Updated: The Surprising New Science That Will Transform Your Sex Life.* New York: Simon & Schuster, 2021.

Orbuch, Iris Kerin, and Amy Stein. *Beating Endo: How to Reclaim Your Life from Endometriosis.* New York: Harper Wave, 2021.

O'Rourke, Meghan. *The Invisible Kingdom: Reimagining Chronic Illness.* New York: Riverhead Books, 2023.

Roberts, Dorothy. *Killing the Black Body: Race, Reproduction, and the Meaning of Liberty.* New York: Vintage Books, 2017.

Ross, Loretta, and Rickie Solinger. *Reproductive Justice: An Introduction*. Oakland: University of California Press, 2017.

Solnit, Rebecca. *The Mother of All Questions*. Chicago: Haymarket Books, 2017.

Taylor, Sonya Renee. *The Body Is Not an Apology: The Power of Radical Self-Love*. Oakland, CA: Berrett-Koehler, 2018.

Tea, Michelle. *Knocking Myself Up: A Memoir of My (In)Fertility*. New York: HarperCollins, 2022.

Tovar, Virgie. *You Have the Right to Remain Fat*. New York: Feminist Press, 2018.

Van der Kolk, Bessel. *The Body Keeps the Score: Brain, Mind, and Body in the Healing of Trauma*. New York: Penguin, 2015.

Weschler, Toni. *Taking Charge of Your Fertility: The Definitive Guide to Natural Birth Control, Pregnancy Achievement and Reproductive Health*. New York: Random House, 2022.

Zapata, Isabel. *In Vitro: On Longing and Transformation*. Minneapolis: Coffee House Press, 2023.

Zucker, Jessica. *I Had a Miscarriage: A Memoir, a Movement*. New York: Feminist Press, 2021.

Notes

1. Introducing a Model of Tracking for Everyone

3   **correctly predicting ovulation.** Sarah Johnson, Lorrae Marriott, and Michael Zinaman, "Can Apps and Calendar Methods Predict Ovulation with Accuracy?" *Current Medical Research and Opinion* 34, no. 9 (May 25, 2018): 1587–1594, https://doi.org/10.1080/03007995.2018.1475348. Further research into the efficacy of menstrual tracking apps is needed.

3   **post-Roe era.** Mark Sherman, "Supreme Court Overturns Roe v. Wade; States Can Ban Abortion," AP News, June 24, 2022, https://apnews.com/article/abortion -supreme-court-decision-854f60302f21c2c35129e58cf8d8a7b0.

3   **delete our tracking apps.** Rina Torchinsky, "How Period Tracking Apps and Data Privacy Fit into a Post–Roe v. Wade Climate," NPR, June 24, 2022, https://www.npr .org/2022/05/10/1097482967/roe-v-wade-supreme-court-abortion-period -apps.

3   **U.S. federal privacy laws.** The Health Insurance Portability and Accountability Act of 1996 (HIPAA) is a federal law that required the creation of national standards to protect sensitive patient health information from being disclosed without the patient's consent or knowledge. Health Insurance Portability and Accountability Act, Pub. L. No. 104–191, § 264, 110 Stat. 1936.

3   **data mining has been able to proliferate.** "FTC Warns Health Apps and Connected Device Companies to Comply with Health Breach Notification Rule," Federal Trade Commission, September 15, 2021, https://www.ftc.gov/news-events/news

/press-releases/2021/09/ftc-warns-health-apps-connected-device-companies
-comply-health-breach-notification-rule; "FTC Finalizes Order with Flo Health, a
Fertility-Tracking App That Shared Sensitive Health Data with Facebook, Google,
and Others," Federal Trade Commission, June 22, 2021, https://www.ftc.gov
/news-events/news/press-releases/2021/06/ftc-finalizes-order-flo-health
-fertility-tracking-app-shared-sensitive-health-data-facebook-google.

4   **rights to abortion.** Mark Sherman, "Supreme Court Overturns Roe v. Wade."

4   **ignored, talked down to, or mistreated.** Maya Dusenbery, *Doing Harm: The
    Truth about How Bad Medicine and Lazy Science Leave Women Dismissed,
    Misdiagnosed, and Sick* (New York: HarperOne, 2018).

4   **blame us for the violence.** Donna Coker et al., "Responses from the Field: Sexual
    Assault, Domestic Violence, and Policing," ACLU Foundation, October 2015, http://
    www.aclu.org/responsesfromthefield.

4   **does not protect us.** Elizabeth A. Armstrong, Miriam Gleckman-Krut, and Lanora
    Johnson, "Silence, Power, and Inequality: An Intersectional Approach to Sexual
    Violence," *Annual Review of Sociology* 44 (May 25, 2018): 99–122, https://doi
    .org/10.1146/annurev-soc-073117-041410.

4   **the language we need to understand our bodies.** Anthony Izaguirre, "'Don't Say
    Gay' Bill Signed by Florida Gov. Ron DeSantis," AP News, March 28, 2022, https://
    apnews.com/article/florida-dont-say-gay-law-signed-56aee61f075a12663f2599
    0c7b31624d.

5   **twenty-eight-day cycle length.** Jonathan R. Bull et al., "Real-World Menstrual
    Cycle Characteristics of More Than 600,000 Menstrual Cycles," *npj Digital
    Medicine* 2, no. 1 (August 27, 2019), https://doi.org/10.1038/s41746-019
    -0152-7; Laurence A. Cole, Donald G. Ladner, and Francis W. Byrn, "The Normal
    Variabilities of the Menstrual Cycle," *Fertility and Sterility* 91, no. 2 (February
    2009): 522–527, https://doi.org/10.1016/j.fertnstert.2007.11.073.

5   **and cycle variability.** Jessica A. Grieger and Robert J. Norman, "Menstrual Cycle
    Length and Patterns in a Global Cohort of Women Using a Mobile Phone App:
    Retrospective Cohort Study," *Journal of Medical Internet Research* 22, no. 6
    (June 24, 2020), https://doi.org/10.2196/17109; Karen C. Schliep et al.,
    "Perceived Stress, Reproductive Hormones, and Ovulatory Function," *Epidemiology*
    26, no. 2 (March 2015): 177–184, https://doi.org/10.1097/ede.0000000
    000000238.

7 **signifier of overall health.** "ACOG Committee Opinion No. 651: Menstruation in Girls and Adolescents: Using the Menstrual Cycle as a Vital Sign," *Obstetrics & Gynecology* 126, no. 6 (December 2015): e143–e146, https://doi.org/10.1097 /aog.0000000000001215.

7 **the mindfulness skill of non-judgmental awareness.** Note that the secular version of mindfulness used in Western psychology and in this book is not the cultural or spiritual Buddhist practice of mindfulness. We've used the therapeutic framework of mindfulness-based stress reduction, an evidence-based practice developed by Jon Kabat-Zinn in the 1970s, as the foundation for our guided exercises. Jon Kabat-Zinn, *Full Catastrophe Living (Revised Edition): Using the Wisdom of Your Body and Mind to Face Stress, Pain, and Illness* (New York: Bantam Books, 2013); Paul Grossman et al., "Mindfulness-Based Stress Reduction and Health Benefits: A Meta-Analysis," *Journal of Psychosomatic Research* 57, no. 1 (July 2004): 35–43, https://doi .org/10.1016/s0022-3999(03)00573-7.

7 **We practice body neutrality.** Anne Poirier, certified intuitive eating counselor and eating disorder specialist, is credited with popularizing the framework of "body neutrality" in a lecture in 2015. Body neutrality took off as the body positivity movement seemed to falter. The body positivity movement began as part of fat-acceptance and fat-liberation efforts with the empowering idea that "all bodies are good bodies." As this message seemed to change as the movement became more popular, body justice activists like Virgie Tovar and Jessamyn Stanley began discussing the commodification of body positivity and its lack of intersectionality. Both engaged in conversations about the language of body neutrality to create ways for people to relate to their bodies without pressure, judgment, or the feeling that their bodies needed to fit into a wellness space, while also highlighting a preference for the radical acceptance and liberation movements. The body neutrality movement continues to be shaped by activists and advocates working to support all bodies in their value. Bethany C. Meyers is one of many who uses their voice and platform to share ways to adapt body neutrality to feel better. Anne Poirier, *The Body Joyful: My Journey from Self-Loathing to Self-Acceptance* (Norwalk: Woodhall Press, 2021); Jessamyn Stanley, *Yoke: My Yoga of Self-Acceptance* (New York: Workman Publishing, 2021); Virgie Tovar, *You Have the Right to Remain Fat* (New York: Feminist Press, 2018); Bethany C. Meyers, The Become Project, September 1, 2023, https://thebecomeproject.com/.

7 **and embodied safety.** Dr. Peter A. Levine is a pioneer of the modern somatics movement in working with trauma. He created the therapeutic intervention Somatic

Experiencing in the 1970s and is sometimes credited with the framework of "safety"—a pathway to working with difficult traumatic stress response. Clinicians and advocates like Pat Ogden and Staci Haines continue to develop this idea and subsequent therapeutic interventions to help combat the often painful impacts of trauma. Peter Payne, Peter A. Levine, and Mardi A. Crane-Godreau, "Somatic Experiencing: Using Interoception and Proprioception as Core Elements of Trauma Therapy," *Frontiers in Psychology* 6 (February 4, 2015), https://doi.org/10.3389/fpsyg.2015.00093; Pat Ogden et al., *Sensorimotor Psychotherapy Interventions for Trauma and Attachment* (New York: Norton, 2015); Staci Haines, *Healing Sex: A Mind-Body Approach to Healing Sexual Trauma* (San Francisco: Cleis Press, 2007).

8   **in extreme cases, legally used.** Rina Torchinsky, "How Period Tracking Apps and Data Privacy Fit into a Post–Roe v. Wade Climate," National Public Radio, June 24, 2022; Emily Baker-White and Sarah Emerson, "Facebook Gave Nebraska Cops a Teen's DMs. They Used Them to Prosecute Her for Having an Abortion," *Forbes*, August 8, 2022.

3. Tracking Defined

18   **history of systematized discrimination.** Loretta Ross and Rickie Solinger, *Reproductive Justice: An Introduction* (Berkeley: University of California Press, 2017); "Sister Song," Sister Song: Women of Color Reproductive Justice Collective, 1994, http://www.sistersong.net/.

18   **worldwide lack of providers.** *Global Strategy on Human Resources for Health: Workforce 2030* (Geneva: World Health Organization, 2016).

18   **to diagnose themselves.** Maya Dusenbery, *Doing Harm: The Truth about How Bad Medicine and Lazy Science Leave Women Dismissed, Misdiagnosed, and Sick* (New York: HarperOne, 2018).

18   **her book *In Vitro*.** Isabel Zapata and Robin Myers, *In Vitro: On Longing and Transformation* (Minneapolis: Coffee House Press, 2023), 32.

19   **something "bad" might happen.** Sally M. Winston and Martin N. Seif, *Overcoming Unwanted Intrusive Thoughts: A CBT-Based Guide to Getting Over Frightening, Obsessive, or Disturbing Thoughts* (Oakland, CA: New Harbinger, 2017).

20   **our own anatomy.** Rachel E. Gross, *Vagina Obscura: An Anatomical Voyage* (New York: Norton, 2023).

28 **interactive mindfulness exercises.** Paul Grossman et al., "Mindfulness-Based Stress Reduction and Health Benefits: A Meta-Analysis," *Journal of Psychosomatic Research* 57, no. 1 (July 2004): 35–43, https://doi.org/10.1016/s0022-3999(03)00573-7.

4. Interconnected Self

31 **systems are all interrelated.** Julius Ohrnberger, Eleonora Fichera, and Matt Sutton, "The Relationship between Physical and Mental Health: A Mediation Analysis," *Social Science & Medicine* 195 (December 2017): 42–49, https://doi.org/10.1016/j.socscimed.2017.11.008.

31 **In this way, countless studies.** Glenn N. Levine et al., "Psychological Health, Well-Being, and the Mind-Heart-Body Connection: A Scientific Statement from the American Heart Association," *Circulation* 143, no. 10 (March 9, 2021), https://doi.org/10.1161/cir.0000000000000947; J. Sundquist et al., "Depression as a Predictor of Hospitalization Due to Coronary Heart Disease," *American Journal of Preventive Medicine* 29, no. 5 (December 2005): 428–433, https://doi.org/10.1016/j.amepre.2005.08.002; Tarani Chandola, Eric Brunner, and Michael Marmot, "Chronic Stress at Work and the Metabolic Syndrome: Prospective Study," *British Medical Journal* 332, no. 7540 (January 20, 2006): 521–525, https://doi.org/10.1136/bmj.38693.435301.80; Gary M. Cooney et al., "Exercise for Depression," *Cochrane Database of Systematic Reviews* 2013, no. 9 (September 12, 2013), https://doi.org/10.1002/14651858.cd004366.pub6.

34 **worth hundreds of billions.** Pamela N. Danzinger, "6 Trends Shaping the Future of the $532B Beauty Business." Forbes, October 12, 2022, https://www.forbes.com/sites/pamdanziger/2019/09/01/6-trends-shaping-the-future-of-the-532b-beauty-business.

38 **around 80 percent.** Pietro Invernizzi et al., "Female Predominance and X Chromosome Defects in Autoimmune Diseases," *Journal of Autoimmunity* 33, no. 1 (August 2009): 12–16, https://doi.org/10.1016/j.jaut.2009.03.005; Fariha Angum et al., "The Prevalence of Autoimmune Disorders in Women: A Narrative Review," *Cureus*, May 13, 2020, https://doi.org/10.7759/cureus.8094.

38 **these conditions can impact every part.** Elinor Cleghorn, *Unwell Women: Misdiagnosis and Myth in a Man-Made World* (New York: Dutton, 2022).

38 **and thyroid disease.** Melanie H. Jacobson et al., "Thyroid Hormones and Menstrual Cycle Function in a Longitudinal Cohort of Premenopausal Women," *Paediatric and Perinatal Epidemiology* 32, no. 3 (March 8, 2018): 225–234, https://doi.org/10.1111/ppe.12462.

40 **experiences such as . . . anxiety.** JoAnn V. Pinkerton, Christine J. Guico-Pabia, and Hugh S. Taylor, "Menstrual Cycle-Related Exacerbation of Disease," *American Journal of Obstetrics and Gynecology* 202, no. 3 (March 2010): 221–231, https://doi.org/10.1016/j.ajog.2009.07.061.

40–41 **obsessive-compulsive disorder (OCD).** Elizabeth M. Mulligan et al., "Effects of Menstrual Cycle Phase on Associations between the Error-Related Negativity and Checking Symptoms in Women," *Psychoneuroendocrinology* 103 (May 2019): 233–240, https://doi.org/10.1016/j.psyneuen.2019.01.027.

41 **post-traumatic stress disorder (PTSD).** Nina M. Carroll and Amy Banks, "Health Care for Female Trauma Survivors (With Posttraumatic Stress Disorder or Similarly Severe Symptoms)," November 4, 2022, https://www.uptodate.com/contents/health-care-for-female-trauma-survivors-with-posttraumatic-stress-disorder-or-similarly-severe-symptoms.

41 **borderline personality disorder.** Tory A. Eisenlohr-Moul et al., "Ovarian Hormones and Borderline Personality Disorder Features: Preliminary Evidence for Interactive Effects of Estradiol and Progesterone," *Biological Psychology* 109 (July 2015): 37–52, https://doi.org/10.1016/j.biopsycho.2015.03.016.

41 **a shift in many symptoms.** Rotem Dan et al., "Sex Differences during Emotion Processing Are Dependent on the Menstrual Cycle Phase," *Psychoneuroendocrinology* 100 (2019): 85–95, https://doi.org/10.1016/j.psyneuen.2018.09.032.

42 **The concept of the "embodied brain."** Julian Kiverstein and Mark Miller, "The Embodied Brain: Towards a Radical Embodied Cognitive Neuroscience," *Frontiers in Human Neuroscience* 9 (May 6, 2015), https://doi.org/10.3389/fnhum.2015.00237.

42 **variability in your cognition.** Siti Atiyah Ali, Tahamina Begum, and Faruque Reza, "Hormonal Influences on Cognitive Function," *Malaysian Journal of Medical Sciences* 25, no. 4 (2018): 31–41, https://doi.org/10.21315/mjms2018.25.4.3.

44 **a big influence on sexuality.** Urszula M. Marcinkowska et al., "Variation in Sociosexuality across Natural Menstrual Cycles: Associations with Ovarian

Hormones and Cycle Phase," *Evolution and Human Behavior* 42, no. 1 (January 2021): 35–42, https://doi.org/10.1016/j.evolhumbehav.2020.06.008.

44 ***Refusing Compulsory Sexuality.*** Sherronda J. Brown, Hess Love, and Grace B. Freedom, *Refusing Compulsory Sexuality: A Black Asexual Lens on Our Sex-Obsessed Culture* (Berkeley, CA: North Atlantic Books, 2022), 7, 147.

45 **tends to decrease sexual arousal.** Urszula M. Marcinkowska et al., "Hormonal Underpinnings of the Variation in Sexual Desire, Arousal and Activity throughout the Menstrual Cycle—A Multifaceted Approach," *Journal of Sex Research* 60, no. 9 (August 26, 2022): 1297–1303, https://doi.org/10.1080/00224499.2022.2110558.

46 **physical and emotional closeness.** Shauna G. Simon et al., "Taking Context to Heart: Momentary Emotions, Menstrual Cycle Phase, and Cardiac Autonomic Regulation," *Psychophysiology* 58, no. 4 (April 16, 2021), https://doi.org/10.1111/psyp.13765.

48 **65 percent of health outcomes.** Carlyn M. Hood, Keith P. Gennuso, Geoffrey Swain, and Bridget B. Catlin, "County Health Rankings," *American Journal of Preventive Medicine* 50, no. 2 (February 1, 2016): 129–135, https://doi.org/10.1016/j.amepre.2015.08.024.

48 **a series of intersecting systems.** The reproductive justice movement, helmed by Sister Song, recognizes systemic harm while supporting a pathway to change. The tenets of the reproductive justice movement (the human right to own our bodies and control our future, the human right to have children, the human right to not have children, and the human right to parent our children in safe and sustainable communities) are foundational to this work. Sister Song: Women of Color Reproductive Justice Collective, 1994, http://www.sistersong.net/.

49 **micro and macro systems around you.** The ecomap, genogram, and culturagram are interactive methods of understanding a person in systems. Ransford Danso, "An Integrated Framework of Critical Cultural Competence and Anti-Oppressive Practice for Social Justice Social Work Research," *Qualitative Social Work* 14, no. 4 (November 12, 2014): 572–588, https://doi.org/10.1177/1473325014558664.

5. Pleasure

52 **Alta Starr, quoted in *Pleasure Activism*.** adrienne maree brown, *Pleasure Activism: The Politics of Feeling Good* (Edinburgh: AK Press, 2019), 386.

52 **Alana Devich Cyril.** adrienne maree brown, *Pleasure Activism: The Politics of Feeling Good*, 311.

56 **why we might have some of the beliefs that we do.** Two tenets of the psychodynamic approach are discussion of past experience (developmental focus) and identification of recurring themes and patterns. This evidence-based intervention has positive outcomes for patient well-being. Jonathan Shedler, "The Efficacy of Psychodynamic Psychotherapy," *American Psychologist* 65, no. 2 (January 1, 2010): 98–109, https://doi.org/10.1037/a0018378.

6. Safety

61 **Trauma can rob us of our sense of safety.** Bessel A. van der Kolk, "The Body Keeps the Score: Memory and the Evolving Psychobiology of Posttraumatic Stress," *Harvard Review of Psychiatry* 1, no. 5 (January 1, 1994): 253–265, https://doi.org/10.3109/10673229409017088.

61 **Where trauma dysregulates, safety regulates.** "Once your external safety has been handled, safety becomes an inside job. You can develop a sense of internal safety, a way of feeling in your body that lets you know you are okay and that everything is all right." Staci Haines, *Healing Sex: A Mind-Body Approach to Healing Sexual Trauma* (San Francisco: Cleis Press, 2007), 5.

63 **Another way to feel safe.** Body neutrality activists like Bethany C. Meyers advocate a building of respect for our body, all the while recognizing that we are more than *just* that body. Bethany C. Meyers, The Become Project, September 1, 2023, https://thebecomeproject.com/.

67 **flooded by a trauma response.** Bessel van der Kolk, *The Body Keeps the Score: Brain, Mind, and Body in the Healing of Trauma* (New York: Penguin, 2014).

67 **come back into ourselves.** Haines, *Healing Sex: A Mind-Body Approach to Healing Sexual Trauma*.

7. Dissociation

73 **This was nothing new.** Amanda Montei, "When I Became a Mother, I Lost My Body—and Realized It Never Belonged to Me," *The Guardian*, September 11, 2023.

73　**primed for consumption.** Amanda Montei, *Touched Out: Motherhood, Misogyny, Consent, and Control* (Boston: Beacon Press, 2023), 2.

74　**Sex educator and activist Staci Haines.** Staci K. Haines, *The Politics of Trauma: Somatics, Healing, and Social Justice* (Berkeley, CA: North Atlantic Books, 2019), 99–122.

76　**over- and underdiagnosed.** Sarah Fay, *Pathological: The True Story of Six Misdiagnoses* (San Francisco: HarperOne, 2023).

78　**some of the top causes.** Emily J. Ozer et al., "Predictors of Posttraumatic Stress Disorder and Symptoms in Adults: A Meta-Analysis," *Psychological Bulletin* 129, no. 1 (January 1, 2003): 52–73, https://doi.org/10.1037/0033-2909.129.1.52; Kathleen C. Basile and Stephen G. Smith, "Sexual Violence Victimization of Women," *American Journal of Lifestyle Medicine* 5, no. 5 (June 3, 2011): 407–417, https://doi.org/10.1177/1559827611409512.

79　**wish for perimenopause to start.** Heather Corinna, *What Fresh Hell Is This? Perimenopause, Menopause, Other Indignities and You* (London: Piatkus, 2021), 18–19.

81　**Mindfulness can help.** Gina R. Silverstein et al., "Effects of Mindfulness Training on Body Awareness to Sexual Stimuli," *Psychosomatic Medicine* 73, no. 9 (November 2011): 817–825, https://doi.org/10.1097/psy.0b013e318234e628.

81　**seek help at lower rates.** Shae M. Nester, Sarah L. Hawkins, and Bethany L. Brand, "Barriers to Accessing and Continuing Mental Health Treatment among Individuals with Dissociative Symptoms," *European Journal of Psychotraumatology* 13, no. 1 (February 17, 2022), https://doi.org/10.1080/20008198.2022.2031594.

81　**increased risk of developing PTSD.** Kimberly B. Werner and Michael G. Griffin, "Peritraumatic and Persistent Dissociation as Predictors of PTSD Symptoms in a Female Cohort," *Journal of Traumatic Stress* 25, no. 4 (July 25, 2012): 401–407, https://doi.org/10.1002/jts.21725.

8. Pain

89　**Where was my voice[?].** Anushay Hossain, *The Pain Gap: How Sexism and Racism in Healthcare Kill Women* (New York: Simon Element, 2022), xvi.

89   **not believing those people as much as they believe others.** Maya Dusenbery, *Doing Harm: The Truth about How Bad Medicine and Lazy Science Leave Women Dismissed, Misdiagnosed, and Sick* (New York: HarperOne, 2018); Karen L. Calderone, "The Influence of Gender on the Frequency of Pain and Sedative Medication Administered to Postoperative Patients," *Sex Roles* 23, no. 11–12 (December 1, 1990): 713–725, https://doi.org/10.1007/bf00289259.

89   **generally lack in-depth knowledge about our bodies.** Dusenbery, *Doing Harm: The Truth about How Bad Medicine and Lazy Science Leave Women Dismissed, Misdiagnosed, and Sick.*

89   **doesn't know as much about them.** Dusenbery, *Doing Harm: The Truth about How Bad Medicine and Lazy Science Leave Women Dismissed, Misdiagnosed, and Sick.*

90   **higher rates than other patients.** Nancy N. Maserejian et al., "Disparities in Physicians' Interpretations of Heart Disease Symptoms by Patient Gender: Results of a Video Vignette Factorial Experiment," *Journal of Women's Health* 18, no. 10 (October 1, 2009): 1661–1667, https://doi.org/10.1089/jwh.2008.1007; Esther H. Chen et al., "Gender Disparity in Analgesic Treatment of Emergency Department Patients with Acute Abdominal Pain," *Academic Emergency Medicine* 15, no. 5 (May 1, 2008): 414–418, https://doi.org/10.1111/j.1553-2712.2008.00100.x; National Pain Report, *Women in Pain Report Significant Gender Bias*, June 1, 2022, https://nationalpainreport.com/women-in-pain-report-significant-gender-bias-8824696.html.

90   **less frequently and at lower doses.** Maserejian et al., "Disparities in Physicians' Interpretations of Heart Disease Symptoms by Patient Gender: Results of a Video Vignette Factorial Experiment"; Chen et al., "Gender Disparity in Analgesic Treatment of Emergency Department Patients with Acute Abdominal Pain"; National Pain Report, *Women in Pain Report Significant Gender Bias*; Dusenbery, *Doing Harm: The Truth about How Bad Medicine and Lazy Science Leave Women Dismissed, Misdiagnosed, and Sick.*

90   **a person's overall well-being.** Sara R. Till, Sawsan As-Sanie, and Andrew Schrepf, "Psychology of Chronic Pelvic Pain: Prevalence, Neurobiological Vulnerabilities, and Treatment," *Clinical Obstetrics and Gynecology* 62, no. 1 (March 1, 2019): 22–36, https://doi.org/10.1097/grf.0000000000000412.

91   **on a scale of 1 to 10.** Joel Katz and Ronald Melzack, "Measurement of Pain," *Surgical Clinics of North America* 79, no. 2 (April 1, 1999): 231–252, https://doi .org/10.1016/s0039-6109(05)70381-9.

91   **alternative pain questionnaire.** Deborah Coady and Nancy Fish, *Healing Painful Sex: A Woman's Guide to Confronting, Diagnosing, and Treating Sexual Pain* (Berkeley, CA: Seal Press, 2011), 107–108.

91   *Healing Painful Sex.* Coady and Fish, *Healing Painful Sex: A Woman's Guide to Confronting, Diagnosing, and Treating Sexual Pain*.

97   **a challenge in diagnosis and understanding.** Sandra Hilton and Carolyn Vandyken, "The Puzzle of Pelvic Pain—A Rehabilitation Framework for Balancing Tissue Dysfunction and Central Sensitization, I," *Journal of Women's & Pelvic Health Physical Therapy* 35, no. 3 (September 1, 2011): 103–113, https://doi .org/10.1097/jwh.0b013e31823b0750; Amélie Levesque et al., "Clinical Criteria of Central Sensitization in Chronic Pelvic and Perineal Pain (Convergences PP Criteria): Elaboration of a Clinical Evaluation Tool Based on Formal Expert Consensus," *Pain Medicine* 19, no. 10 (March 7, 2018): 2009–2015, https://doi .org/10.1093/pm/pny030; Iris Kerin Orbuch and Amy Stein, *Beating Endo: How to Reclaim Your Life from Endometriosis* (New York: Harper Wave, 2021).

100   **complex regional pain syndromes.** Coady and Fish, *Healing Painful Sex: A Woman's Guide to Confronting, Diagnosing, and Treating Sexual Pain*, 182.

104   **They are pretty common.** Qiwei Yang et al., "Comprehensive Review of Uterine Fibroids: Developmental Origin, Pathogenesis, and Treatment," *Endocrine Reviews* 43, no. 4 (November 6, 2021): 678–719, https://doi.org/10.1210/endrev /bnab039; Katherine E. Hartmann et al., "Evidence Summary," Management of Uterine Fibroids—NCBI Bookshelf, December 1, 2017, https://www.ncbi.nlm.nih .gov/books/NBK537747/.

105   **people of color.** Ashley M. Florence and Mary Fatehi, "Leiomyoma," StatPearls— NCBI Bookshelf, July 17, 2023, https://www.ncbi.nlm.nih.gov/books/NBK538273/; Yang et al., "Comprehensive Review of Uterine Fibroids: Developmental Origin, Pathogenesis, and Treatment."

105   **80 percent of uteruses.** Yang et al., "Comprehensive Review of Uterine Fibroids: Developmental Origin, Pathogenesis, and Treatment"; Hartmann et al., "Evidence Summary."

9. Cycle Phases

111 **1.8 billion people.** Aishwarya Rohatgi and Sambit Dash, "Period Poverty and Mental Health of Menstruators during COVID-19 Pandemic: Lessons and Implications for the Future," *Frontiers in Global Women's Health* 4 (March 1, 2023), https://doi.org/10.3389/fgwh.2023.1128169.

113 **outdated, oversimplified averages.** L. Worsfold et al., "Period Tracker Applications: What Menstrual Cycle Information Are They Giving Women?," *Women's Health* 17 (January 1, 2021), https://doi.org/10.1177/17455065211049905; Jonathan Bull et al., "Real-World Menstrual Cycle Characteristics of More Than 600,000 Menstrual Cycles," *NPJ Digital Medicine* 2, no. 1 (August 27, 2019), https://doi.org/10.1038/s41746-019-0152-7; Jessica A. Grieger and Robert J. Norman, "Menstrual Cycle Length and Patterns in a Global Cohort of Women Using a Mobile Phone App: Retrospective Cohort Study," *Journal of Medical Internet Research* 22, no. 6 (June 24, 2020): e17109, https://doi.org/10.2196/17109.

10. Hormones

115 **linked to changes in mood.** Bethany Sander and Jennifer Gordon, "Menstrual Cycle Changes in Estradiol, Stress Reactivity, and Emotion Recognition," *Psychoneuroendocrinology* 153 (July 2023), https://doi.org/10.1016/j.psyneuen.2023.106179.

117 **fifty active hormones.** "Overview of the Endocrine System," U.S. Environmental Protection Agency, February 22, 2024, https://www.epa.gov/endocrine-disruption/overview-endocrine-system.

120 **shown to impact mood.** Simone Toffoletto et al., "Emotional and Cognitive Functional Imaging of Estrogen and Progesterone Effects in the Female Human Brain: A Systematic Review," *Psychoneuroendocrinology* 50 (December 1, 2014): 28–52, https://doi.org/10.1016/j.psyneuen.2014.07.025.

120 **build new bone.** V. Seifert-Klauss et al., "Progesterone and Bone: A Closer Link Than Previously Realized," *Climacteric: The Journal of the International Menopause Society* 15, no. S1 (March 20, 2012): 26–31, https://doi.org/10.3109/13697137.2012.669530.

120 **brain function and memory.** Alison Berent-Spillson et al., "Distinct Cognitive Effects of Estrogen and Progesterone in Menopausal Women," *Psychoneuroendocrinology* 59 (September 1, 2015): 25–36, https://doi .org/10.1016/j.psyneuen.2015.04.020.

120 **affect gastrointestinal function.** Mohammad Alqudah et al., "Progesterone Inhibitory Role on Gastrointestinal Motility," *Physiological Research* 71, no. 2 (April 30, 2022): 193–198, https://doi.org/10.33549/physiolres.934824.

120 **Reduced levels of progesterone.** Karl R. Hansen et al., "Midluteal Progesterone: A Marker of Treatment Outcomes in Couples with Unexplained Infertility," *Journal of Clinical Endocrinology & Metabolism* 103, no. 7 (May 14, 2018): 2743–2751, https://doi.org/10.1210/jc.2018-00642; Eliane G. M. Sanchez et al., "Low Progesterone Levels and Ovulation by Ultrasound Assessment in Infertile Patients," *JBRA Assisted Reproduction* 20, no. 1 (January 1, 2016), https://doi .org/10.5935/1518-0557.20160004; Howard Carp, "Progestogens and Pregnancy Loss," *Climacteric* 21, no. 4 (March 22, 2018): 380–384, https://doi .org/10.1080/13697137.2018.1436166.

123 **genital and pelvic pain conditions.** Deborah Coady and Nancy Fish, *Healing Painful Sex: A Woman's Guide to Confronting, Diagnosing, and Treating Sexual Pain* (Berkeley, CA: Seal Press, 2011); Iris Kerin Orbuch and Amy Stein, *Beating Endo: How to Reclaim Your Life from Endometriosis* (New York: Harper Wave, 2021).

123 **your digestive system.** Malin Ek et al., "Gastrointestinal Symptoms in Women with Endometriosis and Microscopic Colitis in Comparison to Irritable Bowel Syndrome: A Cross-Sectional Study," *Turkish Journal of Gastroenterology* 32, no. 10 (November 2, 2021): 819–827, https://doi.org/10.5152/tjg.2020.19583.

123 **changes in bowel movements.** Adil E. Bharucha and Brian E. Lacy, "Mechanisms, Evaluation, and Management of Chronic Constipation," *Gastroenterology* 158, no. 5 (April 1, 2020): 1232–1249.e3, https://doi.org/10.1053/j.gastro.2019.12.034.

123 **changes in skin.** Rakhi Singh Raghunath, Zoe C. Venables, and G.W.M. Millington, "The Menstrual Cycle and the Skin," *Clinical and Experimental Dermatology* 40, no. 2 (February 11, 2015): 111–115, https://doi.org/10.1111/ced.12588.

125 **the social stress.** Yujie Meng et al., "Menstrual Attitude and Social Cognitive Stress Influence Autonomic Nervous System in Women with Premenstrual Syndrome," *Stress* 25, no. 1 (January 2, 2022): 87–96, https://doi.org/10.1080/10253890

.2021.2024163; Lindsay T. Fourman and Pouneh K. Fazeli, "Neuroendocrine Causes of Amenorrhea—An Update," *Journal of Clinical Endocrinology & Metabolism* 100, no. 3 (March 1, 2015): 812–824, https://doi.org/10.1210/jc.2014-3344.

125 **impact on breathing quality.** Sabine Oertelt-Prigione, "Immunology and the Menstrual Cycle," *Autoimmunity Reviews* 11, no. 6–7 (May 1, 2012): A486–A492, https://doi.org/10.1016/j.autrev.2011.11.023.

125 **changes in bone health.** Peyman Hadji, Enrico Colli, and Pedro-Antonio Regidor, "Bone Health in Estrogen-Free Contraception," *Osteoporosis International* 30, no. 12 (August 24, 2019): 2391–2400, https://doi.org/10.1007/s00198-019 -05103-6; Vanadin Seifert-Klauss and Jerilynn C. Prior, "Progesterone and Bone: Actions Promoting Bone Health in Women," *Journal of Osteoporosis* 2010 (January 1, 2010): 1–18, https://doi.org/10.4061/2010/845180; Tykeysha Powell-Boone et al., "Menstrual Cycle Affects Bladder Pain Sensation in Subjects with Interstitial Cystitis," *Journal of Urology* 174, no. 5 (November 1, 2005): 1832–1836, https://doi.org/10.1097/01.ju.0000176747.40242.3d.

125 **urinary system health.** Guillaume Legendre et al., "Incontinence Urinaire et Ménopause," *Progrès en Urologie* 22, no. 11 (October 1, 2012): 615–621, https://doi.org/10.1016/j.purol.2012.08.267; Powell-Boone et al., "Menstrual Cycle Affects Bladder Pain Sensation in Subjects with Interstitial Cystitis."

126 **symptoms of asthma.** Maria Matteis et al., "Effects of Sex Hormones on Bronchial Reactivity during the Menstrual Cycle," *BMC Pulmonary Medicine* 14, no. 1 (July 1, 2014), https://doi.org/10.1186/1471-2466-14-108.

126 **linked to varying levels of hormones.** Sabine Oertelt-Prigione, "Immunology and the Menstrual Cycle," *Autoimmunity Reviews* 11, no. 6–7 (May 1, 2012): A486–A492, https://doi.org/10.1016/j.autrev.2011.11.023; Niels Bergemann et al., "Estrogen, Menstrual Cycle Phases, and Psychopathology in Women Suffering from Schizophrenia," *Psychological Medicine* 37, no. 10 (April 24, 2007): 1427–1436, https://doi.org/10.1017/s0033291707000578; Chensihan Huang et al., "Associations of Menstrual Cycle Regularity and Length with Cardiovascular Diseases: A Prospective Study from UK Biobank," *Journal of the American Heart Association* 12, no. 11 (June 6, 2023), https://doi.org/10.1161 /jaha.122.029020; Fariha Angum et al., "The Prevalence of Autoimmune Disorders in Women: A Narrative Review," *Cureus*, May 13, 2020, https://doi .org/10.7759/cureus.8094; Michael Camilleri, "Sex as a Biological Variable in Irritable Bowel Syndrome," *Neurogastroenterology and Motility* 32, no. 7

(January 13, 2020), https://doi.org/10.1111/nmo.13802; Maria Raza Tokatli et al., "Hormones and Sex-Specific Medicine in Human Physiopathology," *Biomolecules* 12, no. 3 (March 7, 2022): 413, https://doi.org/10.3390 /biom12030413; Maunil K. Desai and Roberta Diaz Brinton, "Autoimmune Disease in Women: Endocrine Transition and Risk across the Lifespan," *Frontiers in Endocrinology* 10 (April 29, 2019), https://doi.org/10.3389/fendo.2019.00265; Hadine Joffe and Frances J. Hayes, "Menstrual Cycle Dysfunction Associated with Neurologic and Psychiatric Disorders," *Annals of the New York Academy of Sciences* 1135, no. 1 (June 1, 2008): 219–229, https://doi.org/10.1196 /annals.1429.030.

16. Basal Body Temperature (BBT)

253 **a slight increase in BBT.** Mohaned Shilaih et al., "Modern Fertility Awareness Methods: Wrist Wearables Capture the Changes in Temperature Associated with the Menstrual Cycle," *Bioscience Reports* 38, no. 6 (November 30, 2018), https:// doi.org/10.1042/bsr20171279; Hsiu-Wei Su et al., "Detection of Ovulation, a Review of Currently Available Methods," *Bioengineering & Translational Medicine* 2, no. 3 (May 16, 2017): 238–246, https://doi.org/10.1002/btm2.10058; Kaitlyn Steward and Avais Raja, "Physiology, Ovulation and Basal Body Temperature," *StatPearls*, July 22, 2021, https://pubmed.ncbi.nlm.nih.gov/31536292/.

18. Fertility Choices

267 **In her memoir, . . . Michelle Tea.** Michelle Tea, *Knocking Myself Up: A Memoir of My (In)Fertility* (New York: HarperCollins, 2022), ix.

267 **Rebecca Solnit describes.** Rebecca Solnit, *The Mother of All Questions* (Chicago: Haymarket Books, 2017), 5.

268 **as I am now.** Solnit, *The Mother of All Questions*, 5.

269 **diagnosed with infertility.** "Diagnostic Evaluation of the Infertile Female: A Committee Opinion," *Fertility and Sterility* 103, no. 6 (June 1, 2015): e44–e50, https://doi.org/10.1016/j.fertnstert.2015.03.019.

269 **Infertility screening criteria.** "Definitions of Infertility and Recurrent Pregnancy Loss: A Committee Opinion," *Fertility and Sterility* 99, no. 1 (January 1, 2013): 63, https://doi.org/10.1016/j.fertnstert.2012.09.023; "Infertility Workup for the

Women's Health Specialist," *Obstetrics & Gynecology* 133, no. 6 (June 1, 2019, reaffirmed 2023): e377–e384, https://doi.org/10.1097/aog.000000 0000003271.

270 **public health initiatives.** Pamela K. Kohler, Lisa E. Manhart, and William E. Lafferty, "Abstinence Only and Comprehensive Sex Education and the Initiation of Sexual Activity and Teen Pregnancy," *Journal of Adolescent Health* 42, no. 4 (April 2008): 344–351, https://doi.org/10.1016/j.jadohealth.2007.08.026.

271 **Better health and birth outcomes.** Sheree L. Boulet, Christopher S. Parker, and Hani K. Atrash, "Preconception Care in International Settings," *Maternal and Child Health Journal* 10, no. S1 (May 19, 2006): 29–35, https://doi.org/10.1007 /s10995-006-0091-1.

276 **about a third of pregnancies.** Michael J. Zinaman et al., "Estimates of Human Fertility and Pregnancy Loss," *Fertility and Sterility* 65, no. 3 (March 1, 1996): 503–509, https://doi.org/10.1016/s0015-0282(16)58144-8; Xiaobin Wang et al., "Conception, Early Pregnancy Loss, and Time to Clinical Pregnancy: A Population-Based Prospective Study," *Fertility and Sterility* 79, no. 3 (March 1, 2003): 577–584, https://doi.org/10.1016/s0015-0282(02)04694-0; Allen J. Wilcox et al., "Incidence of Early Loss of Pregnancy," *New England Journal of Medicine* 319, no. 4 (July 28, 1988): 189–194, https://doi.org/10.1056 /nejm198807283190401.

276 **Reproductive psychologist Jessica Zucker.** Jessica Zucker, *I Had a Miscarriage: A Memoir, a Movement* (New York: Feminist Press, 2021), 17–18.

19. Perimenopause

279 **not an illness or progressive disease.** Heather Corinna, *What Fresh Hell Is This?: Perimenopause, Menopause, Other Indignities, and You* (London: Piatkus, 2021), 118.

279 **new, more specific hormonal stages.** The STRAW reproductive stages differentiate the reproductive stage (early reproductive, peak reproductive, and late reproductive), menopausal transition stage (early menopausal transition, late menopausal transition), and the postmenopause stage (early postmenopause and late postmenopause). Sioán D. Harlow et al., "Executive Summary of the Stages of Reproductive Aging Workshop + 10," *Menopause* 19, no. 4 (April 1, 2012): 387–395, https://doi.org/10.1097/gme.0b013e31824d8f40; Nancy

Fugate Woods et al., "Transitioning to the Menopausal Transition: A Scoping Review of Research on the Late Reproductive Stage in Reproductive Aging," *Menopause* 28, no. 4 (January 15, 2021): 447–466, https://doi.org/10.1097/gme.0000000000001707.

280 **with official approximations.** Harlow et al., "Executive Summary of the Stages of Reproductive Aging Workshop + 10."

281 **its clinical definition.** Harlow et al., "Executive Summary of the Stages of Reproductive Aging Workshop + 10"; Kimberly Peacock, "Menopause," StatPearls, December 21, 2023, https://www.ncbi.nlm.nih.gov/books/NBK507826/.

282 **a great many people do.** Corinna, *What Fresh Hell Is This?: Perimenopause, Menopause, Other Indignities, and You*, 16–17.